Medical Journal Memos

Judith K. Myer

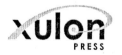
PRESS

*M*edical
*J*ournal
*M*emos

a guide for families with loved ones facing illnesses at
home, in the hospital or long term facilities.

Judith K. Myer

Acknowledgments

It is true that many people touch our lives and so it is in writing a book such as this. I would like to thank and acknowledge those people. First of all, if I had not experienced so very much during the years my daughter, Marla Jeannine Myer, struggled with illness I probably would have been totally oblivious to the true plight of so very many and so to you Marla although death has taken you from this life, this book is possible largely because of you.

To my son Matthew Joseph Myer whose input, probing and sensitivity has allowed me to persevere in this endeavor and for his unending support and understanding when my tunnel vision for this to be published consumed my time.

To my mother, Mary L. Dinsmore, my brother Jerrold R. Mustaine and his wife Nancy J. Mustaine whose support has been unending.

To my dear friends Gail and Ken Radcliffe who have encouraged me and provided thought provoking issues to consider.

To Dr. Arnold L. Schroeter of the Mayo Clinic in Rochester, MN who emanates excellency in caring for his patients needs and who sets a standard by which I gathered input for this publication. To Dr. Joseph E. Levinson of Cincinnati, OH who showed relentless perseverance in caring for his patients. To Edith Shear, an outstanding social worker from Cincinnati, OH who showed me, as she instilled in patients, the knowledge that they have a voice in their own care and should be active participants.

My sincere thanks and gratitude to each and every one for your contributions in making this a reality.

Dedicated to my son,

Matthew Joseph Myer

Who inspires me and whose love
and encouragement are boundless!

and to my daughter,

Marla Jeannine Myer

Who showed great courage in life
and dignity in her death.

Introduction

Congratulations on taking the first step in recording and keeping accurate detailed medical records for yourself and consider keeping one for each of your immediate family members too. This information will be invaluable to you in the future as your life changes with potential new doctors, perhaps relocating, seeking second opinions and more. No longer will you need to "Try To Remember" important dates, medications, procedures, surgeries and more. Additionally, it will expedite the time in filling out medical forms and relaying accurate information to health care providers. Although we all hope we will never be confronted with a medical emergency for ourselves or a loved one, it does happen. Our emotions run high at times like that and it is difficult to recall what may be critical information. Should you or a family member have need to be hospitalized, placed in a nursing facility or rehabilitation center it is nearly impossible to have someone available day and night to stay at bedside. At times such as these, a copy could be placed in your bed tray while a family member will be able to keep one as well. This will help you track your progress, as well as bring questions to mind that you still need answered. It's a great check system for your physician and other health care providers to assess your progress and make recommendations. By keeping this information current it allows you to become an active part of your treatment, not just the person being treated. Although medicine has made great strides and advancements, occasionally a medical tragedy or misdiagnosis does occur. It is not my intention to make this a blueprint for litigation, but should the worst occur to you or a loved one you will be thankful for detailed record keeping. Health care providers keep documented files on you and yet we are usually left with only the option of "trying to remember" what occurred, when and who was involved. Should the worst case scenario occur, a litigation attorney will be thankful for the journal meticulously kept. I pray that it will never be necessary for anything except accurate information to assist you.

TABLE OF CONTENTS

Introduction

Patient Medical information

The Emergency Room

Daily Activities - Week One

Daily Activities - Week Two

Family Health Records

Quarterly Questionnaires

Admissions

Discharges

More Journal Pages

More Expenditures

PRIMARY

MEDICAL

INFORMATION

"Kind words can be short and easy to speak, but their echoes are truly endless."   Mother Teresa

MEDICAL JOURNAL
FOR PATIENTS & FAMILY

Patient's name _____

Patient's address_____

_____

_____

Patient's Phone (   )_____-_____

Emergency Contact Person:_____

Phone Number (   )_____-_____

Relationship:_____

Organ Donor Preference Yes___No___

Blood type_____Pos___Neg___

Name of Primary/Family Doctor:

_____

Phone Number (   )_____-_____

Fax Number   (   )_____-_____

Health Care Plan Provider_____

Health Care Plan Policy No._____

Health Care Plan Phone No. (   )____-_____

Pharmacy Name_____
Pharmacy Phone No. (   )____-____

Prescription known allergies:_____

_____
_____
_____
_____

Current Medications & Dosage_____

_____
_____
_____
_____

Previous Surgeries

Surgery	Doctor	Date
_____	_____	__/__/__
_____	_____	__/__/__
_____	_____	__/__/__
_____	_____	__/__/__
_____	_____	__/__/__
_____	_____	__/__/__
_____	_____	__/__/__
_____	_____	__/__/__
_____	_____	__/__/__
_____	_____	__/__/__
_____	_____	__/__/__
_____	_____	__/__/__
_____	_____	__/__/__

Church/Parish/Synagogue/Mosque
_____

Pastor/Priest/Rabbi_____
Church/Parish/Synagogue/Mosque Address
_____

Church/Parish/Synagogue/Mosque
Phone No (   )____/_____

Employer_____
Phone No. (   )____/____
School (if Minor)_____
Phone No. (   )____/_____   Principal_____

Drivers License No._____
License Plate No._____ State _____

Does the patient have a Will?
Yes_____ No____
Does patient have a Power of Attorney?
Yes_____ No____
Does this include Power of Attorney for Health
Care and a Living Will?
Yes____ No ____
Attorney's name _____
Attorney's Phone No. (   )____/____

THE

EMERGENCY

ROOM

"Hope deferred makes the heart sick, but a longing fulfilled is a tree of life."   *Proverbs 13:12*

The Emergency Room

Date _____ / _____ / _____

Patient name _____

ER doctors's name _____

Triage attendant _____

Method of transportation to hospital:

Car_____   911 Medic_____   Other _____

ER Arrival Time ___:___AM ___:___PM

Released at   ___:___AM ___:___PM

Admission Time ___:___AM ___:___PM

Diagnosis:_____

Temperature ___ Blood Pressure ___/___

Pulse ___   Symptoms _____

_____

Allergy band(if needed)   Yes____No____

Is illness or injury due to an accident?

Yes ___   No ___

If due to accident: Time ___:___AM or PM

Location of accident _____

Witnesses _____

Tests done while in ER _____

_____

_____

_____

Medications/IV's/Blood given while in ER

_____

_____

_____

_____

Attending doctor(s), nurse(s) and comments

_____

_____

_____

_____

Attending aide(s), technician(s) and comments

_____

_____

_____

_____

Requests made by patient or family member(s)

_____

_____

_____

_____

_____

Other observations/comments by the patient or
other family member(s)_____

_____

_____

_____

_____

Known allergies in addition to medications

_____

_____

_____

Where all of your concerns addressed?
Yes___   No___
If not, what?_____

_____

The Emergency Room

Date _____/_____/_____

Patient name _____

ER doctors's name _____

Triage attendant _____

Method of transportation to hospital:

Car_____   911 Medic_____   Other _____

ER Arrival Time ___:___ AM ___:___PM

Released at   ___:___ AM ___:___PM

Admission Time ___:___ AM ___:___PM

Diagnosis:_____

Temperature ___ Blood Pressure ___/___

Pulse ___   Symptoms _____

_____

Allergy band(if needed)   Yes____No_____

Is illness or injury due to an accident?

Yes ___   No ___

If due to accident: Time __:__ AM or PM

Location of accident _____

Witnesses _____

Tests done while in ER_____

_____

_____

_____

Medications/IV's/Blood given while in ER

_____

_____

_____

_____

Attending doctor(s), nurse(s) and comments

_____

_____

_____

_____

Attending aide(s), technician(s) and comments

_____

_____

_____

_____

Requests made by patient or family member(s)

_____

_____

_____

_____

_____

Other observations/comments by the patient or
other family member(s)_____

_____

_____

_____

_____

Known allergies in addition to medications

_____

_____

_____

Where all of your concerns addressed?
Yes___   No___
If not, what?_____

_____

The Emergency Room

Date _____/_____/_____

Patient name _____

ER doctors's name _____

Triage attendant _____

Method of transportation to hospital:

Car_____   911 Medic_____   Other _____

ER Arrival Time ___:___AM ___:___PM

Released at ___:___AM ___:___PM

Admission Time ___:___AM ___:___PM

Diagnosis:_____

Temperature ___ Blood Pressure ___/___

Pulse ___   Symptoms _____

_____

Allergy band(if needed)   Yes_____No_____

Is illness or injury due to an accident?

Yes ___   No ___

If due to accident: Time __:__AM or PM

Location of accident _____

Witnesses _____

Tests done while in ER_____

_____

_____

_____

Medications/IV's/Blood given while in ER

_____

_____

_____

_____

Attending doctor(s), nurse(s) and comments

_____

_____

_____

_____

Attending aide(s), technician(s) and comments

_____

_____

_____

_____

Requests made by patient or family member(s)

_____

_____

_____

_____

_____

Other observations/comments by the patient or
other family member(s)_____

_____

_____

_____

_____

Known allergies in addition to medications

_____

_____

_____

Where all of your concerns addressed?
Yes___ No___
If not, what?_____

_____

The Emergency Room

Date _____ / _____ / _____

Patient name _____

ER doctors's name _____

Triage attendant _____

Method of transportation to hospital:

Car_____ 911 Medic_____ Other _____

ER Arrival Time ___:___AM ___:___PM

Released at ___:___AM ___:___PM

Admission Time ___:___AM ___:___PM

Diagnosis:_____

Temperature ___ Blood Pressure ___/___

Pulse ___ Symptoms _____

_____

Allergy band(if needed) Yes____No____

Is illness or injury due to an accident?

Yes ___ No ___

If due to accident: Time __:__AM or PM

Location of accident _____

Witnesses _____

Tests done while in ER_____

_____

_____

_____

Medications/IV's/Blood given while in ER

_____

_____

_____

_____

Attending doctor(s), nurse(s) and comments

_____

_____

_____

_____

Attending aide(s), technician(s) and comments

_____

_____

_____

_____

15

Requests made by patient or family member(s)

_____
_____
_____
_____
_____

Other observations/comments by the patient or
other family member(s)_____

_____
_____
_____
_____

Known allergies in addition to medications

_____
_____
_____

Where all of your concerns addressed?
Yes___   No___
If not, what?_____

_____

DAILY

ACTIVITIES

WEEK ONE

"The work will wait while you show the child the rainbow, but the rainbow won't wait while you do the work".

Unknown

Activity	Sun _/_/_	Mon _/_/_	Tues _/_/_
Doctors in today and what time			
Tests ordered and why?			
Previous test results			
New Medicines added			
Why new medicines?			
Old Medicines deleted			
Why Medicines deleted?			
Tests performed or Therapy			
Visitors, who and when?			

Additional Comments:

_/_/_

_/_/_

_/_/_

17

| *Wed* | *Thurs* | *Fri* | *Sat* |
_/_/_	_/_/_	_/_/_	_/_/_

<u>**Additional Comments:**</u>
_/_/_
_/_/_
_/_/_

NURSING	7AM-3PM	3PM-11PM	11PM-7AM
SUNDAY DATE / /	T__BP__/__	T__BP__/__	T___BP__/__
MONDAY DATE / /	T___BP__/__	T___BP__/__	T___BP__/__
TUESDAY DATE / /	T___BP__/__	T___BP__/__	T___BP__/__
WEDNESDAY DATE / /	T___BP__/__	T___BP__/__	T___BP__/__
THURSDAY DATE / /	T___BP__/__	T___BP__/__	T___BP__/__
FRIDAY DATE / /	T___BP__/__	T___BP__/__	T___BP__/__
SATURDAY DATE / /	T___BP__/__	T___BP__/__	T___BP__/__

Journal Notes

Journal Notes

Expenditures: Parking/Food/Phone Calls/Miscellaneous

Sunday   Date___/___/___
A. Breakfast_____ Amount$____.____   Comments_____
B. Lunch _____ Amount$____.____   Comments_____
C. Dinner _____ Amount$____.____   Comments_____
D. Parking _____ Amount$____.____   Comments_____
E. Phone _____ Amount$____.____   Comments_____
F. Misc. _____ Amount$____.____   Comments_____

Monday   Date___/___/___
A. Breakfast_____ Amount$____.____   Comments_____
B. Lunch _____ Amount$____.____   Comments_____
C. Dinner _____ Amount$____.____   Comments_____
D. Parking _____ Amount$____.____   Comments_____
E. Phone _____ Amount$____.____   Comments_____
F. Misc. _____ Amount$____.____   Comments_____

Tuesday   Date___/___/___
A. Breakfast_____ Amount$____.____   Comments_____
B. Lunch _____ Amount$·____.____   Comments_____
C. Dinner _____ Amount$____.____   Comments_____
D. Parking _____ Amount$____.____   Comments_____
E. Phone _____ Amount$____.____   Comments_____
F. Misc. _____ Amount$____.____   Comments_____

Wednesday   Date___/___/___
A. Breakfast_____ Amount$____.____   Comments_____
B. Lunch _____ Amount$____.____   Comments_____
C. Dinner _____ Amount$____.____   Comments_____
D. Parking _____ Amount$____.____   Comments_____
E. Phone _____ Amount$____.____   Comments_____
F. Misc. _____ Amount$____.____   Comments_____

Expenditures: Parking/Food/Phone Calls/Miscellaneous

Thursday   Date___/___/___
A. Breakfast_____ Amount$___.___   Comments_____
B. Lunch   _____ Amount$___.___   Comments_____
C. Dinner   _____ Amount$___.___   Comments_____
D. Parking _____ Amount$___.___   Comments_____
E. Phone   _____ Amount$___.___   Comments_____
F. Misc.   _____ Amount$___.___   Comments_____

Friday   Date___/___/___
A. Breakfast_____ Amount$___.___   Comments_____
B. Lunch   _____ Amount$___.___   Comments_____
C. Dinner   ___.__ Amount$___.___   Comments_____
D. Parking _____ Amount$___.___   Comments_____
E. Phone   _____ Amount$___.___   Comments_____
F. Misc.   _____ Amount$___.___   Comments_____

Saturday   Date___/___/___
A. Breakfast_____ Amount$___.___   Comments_____
B. Lunch   _____ Amount$___.___   Comments_____
C. Dinner   _____ Amount$___.___   Comments_____
D. Parking _____ Amount$___.___   Comments_____
E. Phone   _____ Amount$___.___   Comments_____
F. Misc.   _____ Amount$___.___   Comments_____

Additional Comments:

_____
_____
_____
_____
_____
_____

23

DAILY

ACTIVITIES

WEEK TWO

"Of all the properties which belong to honorable men, not one is so highly prized as that of character."   *Henry Clay*

Activity	Sun / /	Mon / /	Tues / /
Doctors in today and what time			
Tests ordered and why?			
Previous test results			
New Medicines added			
Why new medicines?			
Old Medicines deleted			
Why Medicines deleted?			
Tests performed or Therapy			
Visitors, who and when?			

Additional Comments:

/ /
/ /
/ /

24

Wed /_/_	Thurs /_/_	Fri /_/_	Sat /_/_

Additional Comments:

/_/_
/_/_
/_/_

NURSING	7AM-3PM	3PM-11PM	11PM-7AM
SUNDAY ____ DATE / / ___	T__ BP__/___	T__ BP__/__	T___ BP__/__
MONDAY ____ DATE / / ___	T___ BP__/___	T___ BP__/___	T___ BP__/___
TUESDAY ____ DATE / / ___	T___ BP__/___	T___ BP__/___	T___ BP__/___
WEDNESDAY__ DATE / / ___	T___ BP__/___	T___ BP__/___	T___ BP__/___
THURSDAY___ DATE / / ___	T___ BP__/___	T___ BP__/___	T___ BP__/___
FRIDAY ____ DATE / / ___	T___ BP__/___	T___ BP__/___	T___ BP__/___
SATURDAY___ DATE / / ___	T___ BP__/___	T___ BP__/___	T___ BP__/___

Journal Notes

Journal Notes

Expenditures: Parking/Food/Phone Calls/Miscellaneous

Sunday   Date___/___/___
A. Breakfast_____ Amount$___.___   Comments_____
B. Lunch _____ Amount$___.___   Comments_____
C. Dinner _____ Amount$___.___   Comments_____
D. Parking _____ Amount$___.___   Comments_____
E. Phone _____ Amount$___.___   Comments_____
F. Misc. _____ Amount$___.___   Comments_____

Monday   Date___/___/___
A. Breakfast_____ Amount$___.___   Comments_____
B. Lunch _____ Amount$___.___   Comments_____
C. Dinner _____ Amount$___.___   Comments_____
D. Parking _____ Amount$___.___   Comments_____
E. Phone _____ Amount$___.___   Comments_____
F. Misc. _____ Amount$___.___   Comments_____

Tuesday   Date___/___/___
A. Breakfast_____ Amount$___.___   Comments_____
B. Lunch _____ Amount$___.___   Comments_____
C. Dinner _____ Amount$___.___   Comments_____
D. Parking _____ Amount$___.___   Comments_____
E. Phone _____ Amount$___.___   Comments_____
F. Misc. _____ Amount$___.___   Comments_____

Wednesday   Date___/___/___
A. Breakfast_____ Amount$___.___   Comments_____
B. Lunch _____ Amount$___.___   Comments_____
C. Dinner _____ Amount$___.___   Comments_____
D. Parking _____ Amount$___.___   Comments_____
E. Phone _____ Amount$___.___   Comments_____
F. Misc. _____ Amount$___.___   Comments_____

Expenditures: Parking/Food/Phone Calls/Miscellaneous

Thursday Date___/___/___
A. Breakfast_____ Amount$____.____ Comments_____
B. Lunch _____ Amount$____.____ Comments_____
C. Dinner _____ Amount$____.____ Comments_____
D. Parking _____ Amount$____.____ Comments_____
E. Phone _____ Amount$____.____ Comments_____
F. Misc. _____ Amount$____.____ Comments_____

Friday Date___/___/___
A. Breakfast_____ Amount$____.____ Comments_____
B. Lunch _____ Amount$____.____ Comments_____
C. Dinner _____ Amount$____.____ Comments_____
D. Parking _____ Amount$____.____ Comments_____
E. Phone _____ Amount$____.____ Comments_____
F. Misc. _____ Amount$____.____ Comments_____

Saturday Date___/___/___
A. Breakfast_____ Amount$____.____ Comments_____
B. Lunch _____ Amount$____.____ Comments_____
C. Dinner _____ Amount$____.____ Comments_____
D. Parking _____ Amount$____.____ Comments_____
E. Phone _____ Amount$____.____ Comments_____
F. Misc. _____ Amount$____.____ Comments_____

Additional Comments:

_____
_____
_____
_____
_____
_____

DAILY

ACTIVITIES

WEEK THREE

"The way of a fool seems right to him but a wise man listens to advice." **Proverbs 12:15**

Activity	Sun ___/___/___	Mon ___/___/___	Tues ___/___/___
Doctors in today and what time			
Tests ordered and why?			
Previous test results			
New Medicines added			
Why new medicines?			
Old Medicines deleted			
Why Medicines deleted?			
Tests performed or Therapy			
Visitors, who and when?			

Additional Comments:

___/___/___

___/___/___

___/___/___

31

Wed _/_/_	Thurs _/_/_	Fri _/_/_	Sat _/_/_

Additional Comments:

_/_/_

_/_/_

_/_/_

NURSING	7AM-3PM	3PM-11PM	11PM-7AM
SUNDAY ____ DATE / / ___	T__BP__/__	T__BP__/__	T___BP__/__
MONDAY ____ DATE / / ___	T___BP__/__	T___BP__/__	T___BP__/__
TUESDAY ____ DATE / / ___	T___BP__/__	T___BP__/__	T___BP__/__
WEDNESDAY ___ DATE / / ___	T___BP__/__	T___BP__/__	T___BP__/__
THURSDAY ___ DATE / / ___	T___BP__/__	T___BP__/__	T___BP__/__
FRIDAY ____ DATE / / ___	T___BP__/__	T___BP__/__	T___BP__/__
SATURDAY ___ DATE / / ___	T___BP__/__	T___BP__/__	T___BP__/__

Journal Notes

Journal Notes

Expenditures: Parking/Food/Phone Calls/Miscellaneous

Sunday   Date___/___/___
A. Breakfast_____ Amount$____.____   Comments_____
B. Lunch   _____ Amount$____.____   Comments_____
C. Dinner   _____ Amount$____.____   Comments_____
D. Parking _____ Amount$____.____   Comments_____
E. Phone   _____ Amount$____.____   Comments_____
F. Misc.   _____ Amount$____.____   Comments_____

Monday   Date___/___/___
A. Breakfast_____ Amount$____.____   Comments_____
B. Lunch   _____ Amount$____.____   Comments_____
C. Dinner   _____ Amount$____.____   Comments_____
D. Parking _____ Amount$____.____   Comments_____
E. Phone   _____ Amount$____.____   Comments_____
F. Misc.   _____ Amount$____.____   Comments_____

Tuesday   Date___/___/___
A. Breakfast_____ Amount$____.____   Comments_____
B. Lunch   _____ Amount$____.____   Comments_____
C. Dinner   _____ Amount$____.____   Comments_____
D. Parking _____ Amount$____.____   Comments_____
E. Phone   _____ Amount$____.____   Comments_____
F. Misc.   _____ Amount$____.____   Comments_____

Wednesday   Date___/___/___
A. Breakfast_____ Amount$____.____   Comments_____
B. Lunch   _____ Amount$____.____   Comments_____
C. Dinner   _____ Amount$____.____   Comments_____
D. Parking _____ Amount$____.____   Comments_____
E. Phone   _____ Amount$____.____   Comments_____
F. Misc.   _____ Amount$____.____   Comments_____

Expenditures: Parking/Food/Phone Calls/Miscellaneous

Thursday   **Date**___/___/___
A. Breakfast_____ Amount$____.____   Comments_____
B. Lunch _____ Amount$____.____   Comments_____
C. Dinner _____ Amount$____.____   Comments_____
D. Parking _____ Amount$____.____   Comments_____
E. Phone _____ Amount$____.____   Comments_____
F. Misc. _____ Amount$____.____   Comments_____

Friday   **Date**___/___/___
A. Breakfast_____ Amount$____.____   Comments_____
B. Lunch _____ Amount$____.____   Comments_____
C. Dinner _____ Amount$____.____   Comments_____
D. Parking _____ Amount$____.____   Comments_____
E. Phone _____ Amount$____.____   Comments_____
F. Misc. _____ Amount$____.____   Comments_____

Saturday   **Date**___/___/___
A. Breakfast_____ Amount$____.____   Comments_____
B. Lunch _____ Amount$____.____   Comments_____
C. Dinner _____ Amount$____.____   Comments_____
D. Parking _____ Amount$____.____   Comments_____
E. Phone _____ Amount$____.____   Comments_____
F. Misc. _____ Amount$____.____   Comments_____

Additional Comments: _____
_____
_____
_____
_____
_____

DAILY

ACTIVITIES

WEEK FOUR

"A soft answer turneth away wrath; but grievous words stir up anger.:   *Proverbs 15:1*

Activity	Sun _/_/_	Mon _/_/_	Tues _/_/_
Doctors in today and what time			
Tests ordered and why?			
Previous test results			
New Medicines added			
Why new medicines?			
Old Medicines deleted			
Why Medicines deleted?			
Tests performed or Therapy			
Visitors, who and when?			

__Additional Comments:__

_/_/_

_/_/_

_/_/_

Wed _/_/_	**Thurs** _/_/_	**Fri** _/_/_	**Sat** _/_/_

Additional Comments:

_/_/_
_/_/_
_/_/_

NURSING	7AM-3PM	3PM-11PM	11PM-7AM
SUNDAY DATE / /	T__ BP__/__	T__ BP__/__	T__ BP__/__
MONDAY DATE / /	T__ BP__/__	T__ BP__/__	T__ BP__/__
TUESDAY DATE / /	T__ BP__/__	T__ BP__/__	T__ BP__/__
WEDNESDAY DATE / /	T__ BP__/__	T__ BP__/__	T__ BP__/__
THURSDAY DATE / /	T__ BP__/__	T__ BP__/__	T__ BP__/__
FRIDAY DATE / /	T__ BP__/__	T__ BP__/__	T__ BP__/__
SATURDAY DATE / /	T__ BP__/__	T__ BP__/__	T__ BP__/__

Journal Notes

Journal Notes

Expenditures: Parking/Food/Phone Calls/Miscellaneous

Sunday   Date___/___/___
A. Breakfast_____ Amount$____.____   Comments_____
B. Lunch   _____ Amount$____.____   Comments_____
C. Dinner   _____ Amount$____.____   Comments_____
D. Parking _____ Amount$____.____   Comments_____
E. Phone   _____ Amount$____.____   Comments_____
F. Misc.   _____ Amount$____.____   Comments_____

Monday   Date___/___/___
A. Breakfast_____ Amount$____.____   Comments_____
B. Lunch   _____ Amount$____.____   Comments_____
C. Dinner   _____ Amount$____.____   Comments_____
D. Parking _____ Amount$____.____   Comments_____
E. Phone   _____ Amount$____.____   Comments_____
F. Misc.   _____ Amount$____.____   Comments_____

Tuesday   Date___/___/___
A. Breakfast_____ Amount$____.____   Comments_____
B. Lunch   _____ Amount$____.____   Comments_____
C. Dinner   _____ Amount$____.____   Comments_____
D. Parking _____ Amount$____.____   Comments_____
E. Phone   _____ Amount$____.____   Comments_____
F. Misc.   _____ Amount$____.____   Comments_____

Wednesday   Date___/___/___
A. Breakfast_____ Amount$____.____   Comments_____
B. Lunch   _____ Amount$____.____   Comments_____
C. Dinner   _____ Amount$____.____   Comments_____
D. Parking _____ Amount$____.____   Comments_____
E. Phone   _____ Amount$____.____   Comments_____
F. Misc.   _____ Amount$____.____   Comments_____

Expenditures: Parking/Food/Phone Calls/Miscellaneous

Thursday   Date___/___/___
A. Breakfast_____ Amount$____.____   Comments_____
B. Lunch   _____ Amount$____.____   Comments_____
C. Dinner   _____ Amount$____.____   Comments_____
D. Parking   _____ Amount$____.____   Comments_____
E. Phone   _____ Amount$____.____   Comments_____
F. Misc.   _____ Amount$____.____   Comments_____

Friday   Date___/___/___
A. Breakfast_____ Amount$____.____   Comments_____
B. Lunch   _____ Amount$____.____   Comments_____
C. Dinner   _____ Amount$____.____   Comments_____
D. Parking   _____ Amount$____.____   Comments_____
E. Phone   _____ Amount$____.____   Comments_____
F. Misc.   _____ Amount$____.____   Comments_____

Saturday   Date___/___/___
A. Breakfast_____ Amount$____.____   Comments_____
B. Lunch   _____ Amount$____.____   Comments_____
C. Dinner   _____ Amount$____.____   Comments_____
D. Parking   _____ Amount$____.____   Comments_____
E. Phone   _____ Amount$____.____   Comments_____
F. Misc.   _____ Amount$____.____   Comments_____

Additional Comments

_____
_____
_____
_____
_____
_____

44

YOUR

DOCTORS

"A merry heart does good like a medicine; but a broken spirit drieth the bones."   Proverbs 17:22

Follow-up Doctor's Visits

Doctor	*Date*	*Time*

Routine Doctor's Visits

Doctor	_Date/Time_	_New Rx's_

Questions: Asked and Answered

Date   Doctor

__/__/__ _____

Question: _____

_____

_____

_____

Answer: _____

_____

_____

_____

Date   Doctor

__/__/__ _____

Question: _____

_____

_____

_____

Answer: _____

_____

_____

_____

Date   Doctor

__/__/__ _____

Question: _____

_____

_____

_____

Answer: _____

_____

_____

_____

Date   Doctor

__/__/__ _____

Question: _____

_____

_____

_____

Answer: _____

_____

_____

_____

Date   Doctor

__/__/__ _____

Question: _____

_____

_____

_____

Answer: _____

_____

_____

_____

Date   Doctor

__/__/__ _____

Question: _____

_____

_____

_____

Answer: _____

_____

_____

_____

Questions: Asked and Answered

Date   Doctor

__/__/__   _____

Question: _____

_____

_____

_____

Answer: _____

_____

_____

_____

Date   Doctor

__/__/__   _____

Question: _____

_____

_____

_____

Answer: _____

_____

_____

_____

Date   Doctor

__/__/__   _____

Question: _____

_____

_____

_____

Answer: _____

_____

_____

_____

Date   Doctor

__/__/__   _____

Question: _____

_____

_____

_____

Answer: _____

_____

_____

_____

Date   Doctor

__/__/__   _____

Question: _____

_____

_____

_____

Answer: _____

_____

_____

_____

Date   Doctor

__/__/__   _____

Question: _____

_____

_____

_____

Answer: _____

_____

_____

_____

Questions: Asked and Answered

Date   Doctor

__/__/__ _____

Question: _____

_____

_____

_____

Answer: _____

_____

_____

_____

Date   Doctor

__/__/__ _____

Question: _____

_____

_____

_____

Answer: _____

_____

_____

_____

Date   Doctor

__/__/__ _____

Question: _____

_____

_____

_____

Answer: _____

_____

_____

_____

Date   Doctor

__/__/__ _____

Question: _____

_____

_____

_____

Answer: _____

_____

_____

_____

Date   Doctor

__/__/__ _____

Question: _____

_____

_____

_____

Answer: _____

_____

_____

_____

Date   Doctor

__/__/__ _____

Question: _____

_____

_____

_____

Answer: _____

_____

_____

_____

Questions: Asked and Answered

Date   Doctor
__/__/__ _____
Question: _____
_____
_____
_____

Answer: _____
_____
_____
_____

Date   Doctor
__/__/__ _____
Question: _____
_____
_____
_____

Answer: _____
_____
_____
_____

Date   Doctor
__/__/__ _____
Question: _____
_____
_____
_____

Answer: _____
_____
_____
_____

Date   Doctor
__/__/__ _____
Question: _____
_____
_____
_____

Answer: _____
_____
_____
_____

Date   Doctor
__/__/__ _____
Question: _____
_____
_____
_____

Answer: _____
_____
_____
_____

Date   Doctor
__/__/__ _____
Question: _____
_____
_____
_____

Answer: _____
_____
_____
_____

Vitals From Doctors Visits

Doctor   <u>Date</u>   <u>Pulse</u>   <u>BP</u>   <u>Height</u>   <u>Weight</u>   <u>Temp</u>

_____   __/__/__   _____   __/__   _____   _____   _____

<u>Summary:</u>_____

_____

Doctor   <u>Date</u>   <u>Pulse</u>   <u>BP</u>   <u>Height</u>   <u>Weight</u>   <u>Temp</u>

_____   __/__/__   _____   __/__   _____   _____   _____

<u>Summary:</u>_____

_____

Doctor   <u>Date</u>   <u>Pulse</u>   <u>BP</u>   <u>Height</u>   <u>Weight</u>   <u>Temp</u>

_____   __/__/__   _____   __/__   _____   _____   _____

<u>Summary:</u>_____

_____

Doctor   <u>Date</u>   <u>Pulse</u>   <u>BP</u>   <u>Height</u>   <u>Weight</u>   <u>Temp</u>

_____   __/__/__   _____   __/__   _____   _____   _____

<u>Summary:</u>_____

_____

Doctor   <u>Date</u>   <u>Pulse</u>   <u>BP</u>   <u>Height</u>   <u>Weight</u>   <u>Temp</u>

_____   __/__/__   _____   __/__   _____   _____   _____

<u>Summary:</u>_____

_____

Vitals From Doctors Visits

Doctor   Date   Pulse   BP   Height   Weight   Temp
_____   __/__/__   _____   __/__   _____   _____   _____
Summary:_____

_____

Doctor   Date   Pulse   BP   Height   Weight   Temp
_____   __/__/__   _____   __/__   _____   _____   _____
Summary:_____

_____

Doctor   Date   Pulse   BP   Height   Weight   Temp
_____   __/__/__   _____   __/__   _____   _____   _____
Summary:_____

_____

Doctor   Date   Pulse   BP   Height   Weight   Temp
_____   __/__/__   _____   __/__   _____   _____   _____
Summary:_____

_____

Doctor   Date   Pulse   BP   Height   Weight   Temp
_____   __/__/__   _____   __/__   _____   _____   _____
Summary:_____

_____

Vitals From Doctors Visits

Doctor   Date   Pulse   BP   Height   Weight   Temp
_____ _/_/_ _____ _/_ _____ _____ _____
Summary:_____

_____

Doctor   Date   Pulse   BP   Height   Weight   Temp
_____ _/_/_ _____ _/_ _____ _____ _____
Summary:_____

_____

Doctor   Date   Pulse   BP   Height   Weight   Temp
_____ _/_/_ _____ _/_ _____ _____ _____
Summary:_____

_____

Doctor   Date   Pulse   BP   Height   Weight   Temp
_____ _/_/_ _____ _/_ _____ _____ _____
Summary:_____

_____

Doctor   Date   Pulse   BP   Height   Weight   Temp
_____ _/_/_ _____ _/_ _____ _____ _____
Summary:_____

_____

Doctor's Information

Name_____   Phone No (   )____/___
Address_____
Specialty_____   Fax No   (   )____/___

Name_____   Phone No (   )____/__
Address_____
Specialty_____   Fax No   (   )____/___

Name_____   Phone No (   )____/__
Address_____
Specialty_____   Fax No   (   )____/___

Name_____   Phone No (   )____/__
Address_____
Specialty_____   Fax No   (   )____/___

Name_____   Phone No (   )____/__
Address_____
Specialty_____   Fax No   (   )____/___

Name_____   Phone No (   )____/__
Address_____
Specialty_____   Fax No   (   )____/___

Doctor's Information

Name_____   Phone No (   )____/__
Address_____
Specialty_____   Fax No   (   )____/__

Name_____   Phone No (   )____/__
Address_____
Specialty_____   Fax No   (   )____/__

Name_____   Phone No (   )____/__
Address_____
Specialty_____   Fax No   (   )____/__

Name_____   Phone No (   )____/__
Address_____
Specialty_____   Fax No   (   )____/__

Name_____   Phone No (   )____/__
Address_____
Specialty_____   Fax No   (   )____/__

Name_____   Phone No (   )____/__
Address_____
Specialty_____   Fax No   (   )____/__

QUESTIONS

TO ASK...

ASK...

ASK...

"It is easy to be independent when you've got money, but to be independent when you haven't got a thing, that's the Lord's test."　　　*Mahalia Jackson*

NEVER BE AFRAID TO ASK QUESTIONS

ASK ASK ASK ASK ASK ASK ASK ASK

BE INFORMED!

1) *Is the doctor communicating and explaining EVERYTHING to the patient as well as to family members?*

2) *Is what the doctor communicates documented in the patient's charts?*

3) *If you don't understand---are you asking UNDERSTAND UNTIL they explain it to you, so you do? Here are a few questions to consider:*

   A) *What is my diagnosis and what does it mean?*
   B) *Why is a specific test being ordered and what do you anticipate it will show? What will you do if the test is not conclusive?*
   C) *Is there anything I can do to help myself - like diet, etc.?*

4) *If new medications are being prescribed, have ALL possible drug interactions or possible side effects been checked? Have you informed your doctor of any OTC (over the counter) medicine or NATURAL medicine you are taking - better yet, check before taking them! Ask for a pharmacy printout of this available information.*

   A) *Why are you ordering this specific medication over another well known one and what kind of side effects should I be aware of?*
   B) *Are generic prescriptions as safe as name brands?*
   C) *Can any of these prescriptions cause damage to any of my organs?*
   D) *Will this new prescription help me right away?*
   E) *NEVER take another persons prescription medication!*
      ****Know your medicines - your life and that of your loved ones may depend on it!*

ASK   ASK   ASK   ASK   ASK   ASK   ASK

5)   *If the patient is being discharged earlier than what is expected,
ask why...*
   ** Is the release due to medical resolve or prompting from the
   insurance companies?*
   ** If you or the patient disagree, have your concerns against early
   release been documented?*
   ** Did you ask for a copy of the admitting summary and discharge
   summary?*
   ** If you found any errors in these papers, did you bring it to the
   doctor's attention?*
   ** Did you then ask for the corrected summary to be placed in the
   patients chart, as well as a copy of that correction be given to the
   patient or a family member?   *** Did you document this well?*

***** KEEP ALL DOCUMENTATION *****
*****IN A SAFE PLACE*****

6)   *Have you requested (and received) a second opinion? (some
insurances may cover this)*

7)   *Are follow-up appointments scheduled?*

8)   *Do you know your blood type? Have you requested to be typed and
to be given a card to carry with you in your wallet?*

9)   *Do you have allergies and/or serious health conditions? Do you
wear some form of medical alert identification?*

BE OBSERVANT!

1) *Are the doctors, nurses and technicians washing their hands before examining you or your loved one? Are you certain?*
   ***If a sink is not available in your room, there should be sterile gloves or even a waterless sanitizer dispenser available. Their momentary inconvenience might save you, or your loved one, from unnecessary infection. It could also save your life!

2) *Are all doctors, nurses, technicians and therapist ALWAYS checking your name band (if in the hospital or similar facility)to verify you are the person for a particular test, procedure or medication?*
   A) *Consider having someone stay with the patient at night and be an extra set of ears and eyes.*

3) *Are medications being dispensed in a medicine cup or other container? (they should NEVER be handled directly)*
   A) *Know your medications and be sure to question if anyone begins to give you one you are not familiar with, even if it means requesting they show you your chart to verify it to your satisfaction. Don't be afraid to check it out - after all, it is your body.*

4) *Are bio-hazards being disposed of safely and correctly? (this includes more than just contaminated needles)*

5) *Is there an unusually long response time for any calls made to the doctors, nurses or technicians?*
   **If so, did they provide any reason why (such as an unavoidable emergency elsewhere)?
   **Keep in mind that many hospitals are understaffed!

REMEMBER!

1) Keep track of any <u>AND</u> all important documentation together in a safe place!!
    ****This may include anything from copies of test results to copies of questionnaires...
    ****Small home safes are a wonderful place to keep ALL of your important papers, and can be purchased at a nominal price at many office supply and retail stores.

2) Be prepared to see your doctor. Have your questions written down. It is too easy to forget your questions, especially if your doctor is running late. Don't let the doctor hurry you - after all you are important!

3) Be sure to tell your doctor all of your symptoms, no matter how insignificant they may seem to you. A symptom may be a critical part of the puzzle for your correct diagnosis.

4) The doctors, nurses, technicians and other health care workers are human, just like you and me. They might not remember everything, or they might not be able to respond as quickly as you would like. They are the caregivers, so be patient, yet persistent as well.

    Again, just like you and me they have bad days too, but still should maintain an attitude of professionalism. Some will perform their job above and beyond the call of duty, by not only dispensing medical care but by dispensing cheer as well. Take a moment to thank those who go the extra mile or give that extra smile.

FAMILY

HEALTH

RECORDS

"Better a poor man whose walk is blameless than a fool whose lips are perverse."   *Proverbs 19:1*

Family Health Record

	Husband		Wife	

Husband

Name _____

Birth date ___/___/___

Blood Type____Pos___Neg___

Tetanus shot and boosters

_____

_____

_____

Wife

Name_____

Birth date ___/___/___

Blood Type____Pos___Neg__

Tetanus shot and boosters

_____

_____

_____

Child

Name _____

Birth date ___/___/___

Birth weight ____Lb. ____Oz.

Birth length _____inches

Blood Type____Pos___Neg___

Child

Name _____

Birth date ___/___/___

Birth weight ____Lb. ____Oz.

Birth length _____inches

Blood Type____Pos___Neg__

Immunizations

Vaccine	Date	Physician
DPT 1	___/___/___	_____
DPT 2	___/___/___	_____
DPT 3	___/___/___	_____
DPT		
Booster	___/___/___	_____
	___/___/___	_____
Small		
Pox	___/___/___	_____
Polio	___/___/___	_____
Measles	___/___/___	_____
Mumps	___/___/___	_____
TB	___/___/___	_____
Other	___/___/___	_____

Immunizations

Vaccine	Date	Physician
DPT 1	___/___/___	_____
DPT 2	___/___/___	_____
DPT 3	___/___/___	_____
DPT		
Booster	___/___/___	_____
	___/___/___	_____
Small		
Pox	___/___/___	_____
Polio	___/___/___	_____
Measles	___/___/___	_____
Mumps	___/___/___	_____
TB	___/___/___	_____
Other	___/___/___	_____

Family Health Record

Child		Child	

Name _____   **Name** _____

Birth date __/__/__   **Birth date** __/__/__

Birth weight ____Lb. ____Oz.   **Birth weight**____Lb. ____Oz.

Birth length _____inches   **Birth length** _____inches

Blood Type____Pos__Neg__   **Blood Type**____Pos__Neg__

Immunizations   ## Immunizations

Vaccine	*Date*	*Physician*		*Vaccine*	*Date*	*Physician*

DPT 1   __/__/__   _____   DPT 1   __/__/__   _____

DPT 2   __/__/__   _____   DPT 2   __/__/__   _____

DPT 3   __/__/__   _____   DPT 3   __/__/__   _____

DPT   DPT

Booster __/__/__   _____   Booster __/__/__   _____

         __/__/__   _____   __/__/__   _____

Small   Small

Pox   __/__/__   _____   Pox   __/__/__   _____

Polio   __/__/__   _____   Polio   __/__/__   _____

Measles __/__/__   _____   Measles __/__/__   _____

Mumps   __/__/__   _____   Mumps   __/__/__   _____

TB   __/__/__   _____   TB   __/__/__   _____

Other   __/__/__   _____   Other   __/__/__   _____

Distinguishing Birthmarks, Tattoos/Body Piercing for any family member

Name	**Location**	**Description**
_____	_____	_____
_____	_____	_____
_____	_____	_____
_____	_____	_____
_____	_____	_____

Drug Allergies and Reactions

Name of Prescription	Type of Reaction	Date of Reaction
		___/___/___
		___/___/___
		___/___/___
		___/___/___
		___/___/___
		___/___/___
		___/___/___
		___/___/___
		___/___/___
		___/___/___
		___/___/___
		___/___/___
		___/___/___
		___/___/___
		___/___/___
		___/___/___
		___/___/___
		___/___/___
		___/___/___
		___/___/___
		___/___/___
		___/___/___
		___/___/___
		___/___/___
		___/___/___
		___/___/___
		___/___/___
		___/___/___
		___/___/___
		___/___/___
		___/___/___

Drug Allergies and Reactions

Name of Prescription	Type of Reaction	Date of Reaction
		___/___/___
		___/___/___
		___/___/___
		___/___/___
		___/___/___
		___/___/___
		___/___/___
		___/___/___
		___/___/___
		___/___/___
		___/___/___
		___/___/___
		___/___/___
		___/___/___
		___/___/___
		___/___/___
		___/___/___
		___/___/___
		___/___/___
		___/___/___
		___/___/___
		___/___/___
		___/___/___
		___/___/___
		___/___/___
		___/___/___
		___/___/___
		___/___/___
		___/___/___
		___/___/___
		___/___/___

Prescription Ledger

Name of Rx	Dosage	Start Date	Stop Date	Reason for Stopping
		__/__/__	__/__/__	
		__/__/__	__/__/__	
		__/__/__	__/__/__	
		__/__/__	__/__/__	
		__/__/__	__/__/__	
		__/__/__	__/__/__	
		__/__/__	__/__/__	
		__/__/__	__/__/__	
		__/__/__	__/__/__	
		__/__/__	__/__/__	
		__/__/__	__/__/__	
		__/__/__	__/__/__	
		__/__/__	__/__/__	
		__/__/__	__/__/__	
		__/__/__	__/__/__	
		__/__/__	__/__/__	
		__/__/__	__/__/__	
		__/__/__	__/__/__	
		__/__/__	__/__/__	
		__/__/__	__/__/__	
		__/__/__	__/__/__	
		__/__/__	__/__/__	
		__/__/__	__/__/__	
		__/__/__	__/__/__	
		__/__/__	__/__/__	
		__/__/__	__/__/__	
		__/__/__	__/__/__	
		__/__/__	__/__/__	
		__/__/__	__/__/__	

Prescription Ledger

Name of Rx	Dosage	Start Date	Stop Date	Reason for Stopping
		_/_/_	_/_/_	
		_/_/_	_/_/_	
		_/_/_	_/_/_	
		_/_/_	_/_/_	
		_/_/_	_/_/_	
		_/_/_	_/_/_	
		_/_/_	_/_/_	
		_/_/_	_/_/_	
		_/_/_	_/_/_	
		_/_/_	_/_/_	
		_/_/_	_/_/_	
		_/_/_	_/_/_	
		_/_/_	_/_/_	
		_/_/_	_/_/_	
		_/_/_	_/_/_	
		_/_/_	_/_/_	
		_/_/_	_/_/_	
		_/_/_	_/_/_	
		_/_/_	_/_/_	
		_/_/_	_/_/_	
		_/_/_	_/_/_	
		_/_/_	_/_/_	
		_/_/_	_/_/_	
		_/_/_	_/_/_	
		_/_/_	_/_/_	
		_/_/_	_/_/_	
		_/_/_	_/_/_	
		_/_/_	_/_/_	
		_/_/_	_/_/_	
		_/_/_	_/_/_	
		_/_/_	_/_/_	
		_/_/_	_/_/_	

Prescription Ledger

Name of Rx	Dosage	Start Date	Stop Date	Reason for Stopping
		_/_/_	_/_/_	
		_/_/_	_/_/_	
		_/_/_	_/_/_	
		_/_/_	_/_/_	
		_/_/_	_/_/_	
		_/_/_	_/_/_	
		_/_/_	_/_/_	
		_/_/_	_/_/_	
		_/_/_	_/_/_	
		_/_/_	_/_/_	
		_/_/_	_/_/_	
		_/_/_	_/_/_	
		_/_/_	_/_/_	
		_/_/_	_/_/_	
		_/_/_	_/_/_	
		_/_/_	_/_/_	
		_/_/_	_/_/_	
		_/_/_	_/_/_	
		_/_/_	_/_/_	
		_/_/_	_/_/_	
		_/_/_	_/_/_	
		_/_/_	_/_/_	
		_/_/_	_/_/_	
		_/_/_	_/_/_	
		_/_/_	_/_/_	
		_/_/_	_/_/_	
		_/_/_	_/_/_	
		_/_/_	_/_/_	

Prescription Ledger

Name of Rx	Dosage	Start Date	Stop Date	Reason for Stopping
		__/__/__	__/__/__	
		__/__/__	__/__/__	
		__/__/__	__/__/__	
		__/__/__	__/__/__	
		__/__/__	__/__/__	
		__/__/__	__/__/__	
		__/__/__	__/__/__	
		__/__/__	__/__/__	
		__/__/__	__/__/__	
		__/__/__	__/__/__	
		__/__/__	__/__/__	
		__/__/__	__/__/__	
		__/__/__	__/__/__	
		__/__/__	__/__/__	
		__/__/__	__/__/__	
		__/__/__	__/__/__	
		__/__/__	__/__/__	
		__/__/__	__/__/__	
		__/__/__	__/__/__	
		__/__/__	__/__/__	
		__/__/__	__/__/__	
		__/__/__	__/__/__	
		__/__/__	__/__/__	
		__/__/__	__/__/__	
		__/__/__	__/__/__	
		__/__/__	__/__/__	
		__/__/__	__/__/__	
		__/__/__	__/__/__	
		__/__/__	__/__/__	
		__/__/__	__/__/__	
		__/__/__	__/__/__	
		__/__/__	__/__/__	
		__/__/__	__/__/__	
		__/__/__	__/__/__	

Prescription Ledger

Name of Rx	Dosage	Start Date	Stop Date	Reason for Stopping
		__/__/__	__/__/__	
		__/__/__	__/__/__	
		__/__/__	__/__/__	
		__/__/__	__/__/__	
		__/__/__	__/__/__	
		__/__/__	__/__/__	
		__/__/__	__/__/__	
		__/__/__	__/__/__	
		__/__/__	__/__/__	
		__/__/__	__/__/__	
		__/__/__	__/__/__	
		__/__/__	__/__/__	
		__/__/__	__/__/__	
		__/__/__	__/__/__	
		__/__/__	__/__/__	
		__/__/__	__/__/__	
		__/__/__	__/__/__	
		__/__/__	__/__/__	
		__/__/__	__/__/__	
		__/__/__	__/__/__	
		__/__/__	__/__/__	
		__/__/__	__/__/__	
		__/__/__	__/__/__	
		__/__/__	__/__/__	
		__/__/__	__/__/__	
		__/__/__	__/__/__	
		__/__/__	__/__/__	
		__/__/__	__/__/__	
		__/__/__	__/__/__	
		__/__/__	__/__/__	
		__/__/__	__/__/__	
		__/__/__	__/__/__	
		__/__/__	__/__/__	

Prescription Ledger

Name of Rx	Dosage	Start Date	Stop Date	Reason for Stopping
		__/__/__	__/__/__	
		__/__/__	__/__/__	
		__/__/__	__/__/__	
		__/__/__	__/__/__	
		__/__/__	__/__/__	
		__/__/__	__/__/__	
		__/__/__	__/__/__	
		__/__/__	__/__/__	
		__/__/__	__/__/__	
		__/__/__	__/__/__	
		__/__/__	__/__/__	
		__/__/__	__/__/__	
		__/__/__	__/__/__	
		__/__/__	__/__/__	
		__/__/__	__/__/__	
		__/__/__	__/__/__	
		__/__/__	__/__/__	
		__/__/__	__/__/__	
		__/__/__	__/__/__	
		__/__/__	__/__/__	
		__/__/__	__/__/__	
		__/__/__	__/__/__	
		__/__/__	__/__/__	
		__/__/__	__/__/__	
		__/__/__	__/__/__	
		__/__/__	__/__/__	
		__/__/__	__/__/__	
		__/__/__	__/__/__	
		__/__/__	__/__/__	
		__/__/__	__/__/__	
		__/__/__	__/__/__	
		__/__/__	__/__/__	

Non-Prescription Allergies

Foods	You	Other	Relationship	Reaction	Date
Eggs	___	___	_____	_____	/ /
Milk	___	___	_____	_____	/ /
MSG	___	___	_____	_____	/ /
Peanuts	___	___	_____	_____	/ /
Other	___	___	_____	_____	/ /
_____	___	___	_____	_____	/ /
_____	___	___	_____	_____	/ /
_____	___	___	_____	_____	/ /

Indoor-Outdoor

	You	Other	Relationship	Reaction	Date
Dust	___	___	_____	_____	/ /
Grass	___	___	_____	_____	/ /
Mold	___	___	_____	_____	/ /
Pollen	___	___	_____	_____	/ /
Ragweed	___	___	_____	_____	/ /
Other	___	___	_____	_____	/ /
_____	___	___	_____	_____	/ /
_____	___	___	_____	_____	/ /
_____	___	___	_____	_____	/ /

Miscellaneous

	You	Other	Relationship	Reaction	Date
Adhesive tape	___	___	_____	_____	/ /
Bee stings	___	___	_____	_____	/ /
Flu vaccine	___	___	_____	_____	/ /
Iodine	___	___	_____	_____	/ /
Latex	___	___	_____	_____	/ /
Other	___	___	_____	_____	/ /
_____	___	___	_____	_____	/ /
_____	___	___	_____	_____	/ /
_____	___	___	_____	_____	/ /

Do you or a family member have (or had) the following:

Health Issue	Y/N	You	Other	Relationship
Acid Reflux				
Aids				
Alzheimers				
Amnesia				
Anemia				
Angina				
Angioplasty				
Anorexia				
Appendicitis				
Arteriosclerosis				
Arthritis				
Asthma				
Autism				
Bladder disorder				
Bronchitis				
Bulimia				
Bursitis				
Cancer				
Cataract				
Chicken Pox				
Crohns disease				
Cystic fibrosis				
Cystitis				
Croup				

Health Issue	Y/N	You	Other	Relationship
Diabetes				
Diarrhea				
Diphtheria				
Diverticulitis				
Emphysema				
Endrometriosis				
Epilepsy				
Epstein-Barr				
Fainting spells				
Gallstones				
Gastritis				
Glaucoma				
Goiter				
Hearing loss				
Heart attack				
Heart disease				
Heart murmur				
Hemophilia				
Hepatitis				
Hernia				
Iritis				
Irritable bowel				
Jaundice				
Joint replaced				
Kidney disease				
Kidney stones				

Health Issue	Y/N	You	Other	Relationship
Laryngitis	___	___	___	_____
Leukemia	___	___	___	_____
Liver disease	___	___	___	_____
Lockjaw	___	___	___	_____
Lung disease	___	___	___	_____
Lupus	___	___	___	_____
Lyme disease	___	___	___	_____
Malaria	___	___	___	_____
Mastectomy	___	___	___	_____
Measles	___	___	___	_____
Meningitis	___	___	___	_____
Migraine	___	___	___	_____
Mononucleosis	___	___	___	_____
Mumps	___	___	___	_____
Numbness	___	___	___	_____
Otitis media	___	___	___	_____
Pacemaker	___	___	___	_____
Paget's disease	___	___	___	_____
Pancreatitis	___	___	___	_____
Panic disorder	___	___	___	_____
Paralysis	___	___	___	_____
Peptic ulcers	___	___	___	_____
Pneumonia	___	___	___	_____
Polyps	___	___	___	_____
Psoriasis	___	___	___	_____
Rickets	___	___	___	_____

Health Issue	Y/N	You	Other	Relationship
Rubella	____	____	____	_____
Sciatica	____	____	____	_____
Scleroderma	____	____	____	_____
Scoliosis	____	____	____	_____
Seizures	____	____	____	_____
Shingles	____	____	____	_____
Sickle cell	____	____	____	_____
Sinusitis	____	____	____	_____
Sleep apnea	____	____	____	_____
Still birth	____	____	____	_____
Stroke	____	____	____	_____
Thyroid disease	____	____	____	_____
Tinnitus	____	____	____	_____
TMJ syndrome	____	____	____	_____
Tonsillitis	____	____	____	_____
Transfusion	____	____	____	_____
Ulcer	____	____	____	_____
Vertigo	____	____	____	_____

Others

_____	____	____	____	_____
_____	____	____	____	_____
_____	____	____	____	_____
_____	____	____	____	_____
_____	____	____	____	_____
_____	____	____	____	_____

New Symptoms - Does Your Doctor Know?
Symptom and Duration

	Date began	1-3 weeks	1-2 months	Longer
Back pain	__/__/__	_____	_____	_____
Bloody stool	__/__/__	_____	_____	_____
Breast lump	__/__/__	_____	_____	_____
Bruising	__/__/__	_____	_____	_____
Chest pain	__/__/__	_____	_____	_____
Constipation	__/__/__	_____	_____	_____
Cough	__/__/__	_____	_____	_____
Diarrhea	__/__/__	_____	_____	_____
Dizziness	__/__/__	_____	_____	_____
Enlarged glands	__/__/__	_____	_____	_____
Excessive thirst	__/__/__	_____	_____	_____
Fever	__/__/__	_____	_____	_____
Headaches	__/__/__	_____	_____	_____
Heartburn	__/__/__	_____	_____	_____
Hearing loss	__/__/__	_____	_____	_____
Joint pain	__/__/__	_____	_____	_____
Joint swelling	__/__/__	_____	_____	_____
Mole change	__/__/__	_____	_____	_____
Muscle pain	__/__/__	_____	_____	_____
Nose bleeds	__/__/__	_____	_____	_____
Seizures	__/__/__	_____	_____	_____
Sinus problems	__/__/__	_____	_____	_____
Skin rash	__/__/__	_____	_____	_____
Sores (not healing)	__/__/__	_____	_____	_____
Speech change	__/__/__	_____	_____	_____
Stomach pain	__/__/__	_____	_____	_____
Thirst (excessive)	__/__/__	_____	_____	_____
Urination problem	__/__/__	_____	_____	_____
Vision changes	__/__/__	_____	_____	_____
Weight gain	__/__/__	_____	_____	_____
Weight loss	__/__/__	_____	_____	_____

QUARTERLY

QUESTIONNAIRES

"A heart at peace gives life to the body."
Proverbs 14:30

Quarterly Questionnaire Review

(For use in Chronic Disease and Short Term Acute Illness)

Time covered: ___/___/___ through ___/___/___

Patient's name: _____ DOB: ___/___/___

Current age: _____ Gender: Female _____ Male _____

Height ___Ft ___In Weight ___LB

Recent weight gain: Yes___ No ___ Recent weight loss: Yes___ No ___

Family doctor: _____

Has patient had new x-rays in previous three months? Yes ___ No ___
If yes, x-rays requested: _____
_____

Name of facility that performed x-rays: _____
Were there new findings from these x-rays? Yes ___ No ___
New findings: _____
_____
_____

Were other tests or procedures requested in previous three months? Yes ___ No ___
Name of procedures performed: _____

Does patient have copy of reports from x-rays and procedures? Yes ___ No ___

Have you recently traveled outside of the United States? Yes ___ No ___
If yes, did this travel require specific inoculations? Yes ___ No ___
If yes, what ones were required? _____

Did you have any adverse reaction to the inoculations? Yes ___ No ___
If yes, what type of reaction? _____
Date of reaction: ___/___/___ Was treatment needed? Yes ___ No ___
Have you recently received a blood transfusion? Yes ___ No ___
If yes, how many units were required? _____
Did you ever receive blood transfusions before 1980? Yes ___ No ___
between 1980-1990? Yes ___ No ___ , after 1990? Yes ___ No ___

76

Name of **All** medications currently taking prescribed or not - including vitamins, over the counter medications (OTC), herbal or natural therapy, pain relievers, cold medication, laxatives, nutritional supplement (such as Ensure), diuretics or contraceptives:

Medication	_Supplement/Other_	_Dosage_	_How often_
_____	_____	_____	_____
_____	_____	_____	_____
_____	_____	_____	_____
_____	_____	_____	_____
_____	_____	_____	_____
_____	_____	_____	_____
_____	_____	_____	_____
_____	_____	_____	_____
_____	_____	_____	_____
_____	_____	_____	_____
_____	_____	_____	_____

To be completed by FEMALE only:

Have you had a pelvic exam with Pap smear in past 3 months? Yes ___ No ___
If not, have you had one in the past year? Yes ___ No ___
in the past 1-3 years? Yes ___ No ___, 3-5 years? Yes ___ No ___
Has it been more than 5 years? Yes ___ No ___
Have you ever been informed that your Pap smear was abnormal? Yes ___ No ___
Have you had a hysterectomy? Yes ___ No ___ If yes, when? ___/___/___
Age at time? ___ Are you on hormone replacement? Yes ___ No ___

Do you routinely have a mammogram? Yes ___ No ___
When was your last mammogram: within the past 3 months? Yes ___ No ___
Less than 1 year? Yes ___ No ___, 1-2 years? Yes ___ No ___
2-5 years? Yes ___ No ___, Never? Yes ___ No ___
Are your periods regular? Yes ___ No ___ Last period? ___/___/___
Are you taking birth control pills? Yes ___ No ___
Are you currently pregnant? Yes ___ No ___

77

To be completed by MALE only:

Have you ever had a prostate examination?   Yes ___ No ___

If yes, was it in the past 3 months?   Yes ___ No ___

less than 1 year? Yes ____ No ____, 1-2 years?   Yes ___ No ___

over 2 years? Yes ____ No ____, Never?   Yes ___ No ___

Have you ever had an abnormal prostate examination?   Yes ___ No ___

If yes, when? ____ / ____ / ____

Have you ever had a vasectomy?   Yes ___ No ___

If yes, when? ____ / ____ / ____   Age at time? _____

Have you recently been experiencing any of the following:

Symptom	Yes	No	When occurred	Currently
Shortness of breath:	____	____	_____	_____
Excessive coughing:	____	____	_____	_____
Coughed up blood:	____	____	_____	_____
Coughed up sputum:	____	____	_____	_____
Chest pain:	____	____	_____	_____
Chest pressure:	____	____	_____	_____
Tightness in arms:	____	____	_____	_____
Excessive sweating:	____	____	_____	_____
Nausea:	____	____	_____	_____
Heart pounding:	____	____	_____	_____
Blurred vision:	____	____	_____	_____
Double vision:	____	____	_____	_____
Leg or foot swelling:	____	____	_____	_____
Dizziness:	____	____	_____	_____
Weakness:	____	____	_____	_____
Numbness:	____	____	_____	_____
Incontinence:	____	____	_____	_____
Excessive Thirst:	____	____	_____	_____
Depression:	____	____	_____	_____

OTHER

_____	____	____	_____	_____
_____	____	____	_____	_____
_____	____	____	_____	_____

Are you at risk for AIDS or HIV?   Yes____ No____
Have you recently been exposed to any infectious disease?   Yes____ No____

Have you ever smoked? · Yes____ No____ If yes, how many packs per day? __
Do you smoke now?   Yes____ No____
If smoking, is your choice: Cigarettes____ Cigars____ Pipe____ Other_____
Do you drink alcohol? Occasionally____ Socially____ Daily____ Never____

What caffeine do you consume daily? Coffee____   Tea____ Soda Pop____
Total 8 Oz. servings of caffeine daily?   0-2____   3-5____ 6 or more____

Do you routinely exercise?   Daily_____ 2-3 days per week_____
3-5 days per week_____   Never_____

How many servings of fruit do you eat daily?   1-2____ 3-5____ None____
How many servings of vegetables do you eat daily? 1-2____ 3-5____ None____
How many Glasses of water do you drink daily?   1-3____ 4-6____ 7-10____

Have you or any blood relatives ever been diagnosed with cancer?

Type of cancer	You	Other	Treated	Year
Brain cancer	____	____	____	____
Breast cancer	____	____	____	____
Colon cancer	____	____	____	____
Leukemia	____	____	____	____
Lung cancer	____	____	____	____
Ovarian cancer	____	____	____	____
Pancreatic cancer	____	____	____	____
Prostate cancer	____	____	____	____
Rectal cancer	____	____	____	____
Thyroid cancer	____	____	____	____
OTHER				
_____	____	____	____	____
_____	____	____	____	____
_____	____	____	____	____

79

Quarterly Questionnaire Review

(For use in Chronic Disease and Short Term Acute Illness)

Time covered: ___/___/___ through ___/___/___

Patient's name: _____ DOB: ___/___/___
Current age: _____   Gender: Female _____   Male _____
Height ____Ft ____In   Weight _____LB
Recent weight gain: Yes____ No ____   Recent weight loss: Yes____ No ____
Family doctor: _____

Has patient had new x-rays in previous three months?   Yes ____ No ___
If yes, x-rays requested: _____
_____
Name of facility that performed x-rays: _____
Were there new findings from these x-rays?   Yes ____ No____
New findings: _____
_____
_____
Were other tests or procedures requested in previous three months? Yes ___ No___
Name of procedures performed: _____
_____
Does patient have copy of reports from x-rays and procedures? Yes ___ No ____

Have you recently traveled outside of the United States?   Yes ____No____
If yes, did this travel require specific inoculations?   Yes ____No ____
If yes, what ones were required? _____
_____
Did you have any adverse reaction to the inoculations?   Yes ____No ____
If yes, what type of reaction? _____
Date of reaction: ___/___/___ ˙ Was treatment needed? Yes ___ No ___
Have you recently received a blood transfusion?   Yes ___No ___
If yes, how many units were required?   _____
Did you ever receive blood transfusions before 1980?   Yes ___No ____
between 1980-1990? Yes _____ No ____,   after 1990?   Yes ___ No ____

Name of **All** medications currently taking prescribed or not - including vitamins, over the counter medications (OTC), herbal or natural therapy, pain relievers, cold medication, laxatives, nutritional supplement (such as Ensure), diuretics or contraceptives:

Medication	_Supplement/Other_	_Dosage_	_How often_

To be completed by FEMALE only:

Have you had a pelvic exam with Pap smear in past 3 months? Yes ___ No ___
If not, have you had one in the past year? Yes ___ No ___
in the past 1-3 years? Yes ____ No ____, 3-5 years? Yes ___ No ___
Has it been more than 5 years? Yes ____ No ____
Have you ever been informed that your Pap smear was abnormal? Yes ___ No ___
Have you had a hysterectomy? Yes ____ No ____ If yes, when? ___/___/___
Age at time? _____ Are you on hormone replacement? Yes ___ No ___

Do you routinely have a mammogram? Yes ___ No ___
When was your last mammogram: within the past 3 months? Yes ___ No ___
Less than 1 year? Yes ____ No ____, 1-2 years? Yes ___ No ___
2-5 years? Yes ____ No ____, Never? Yes ____ No ____
Are your periods regular? Yes ____ No ____ Last period? ___/___/___
Are you taking birth control pills? Yes ___ No ___
Are you currently pregnant? Yes ___ No ___

To be completed by MALE only:

Have you ever had a prostate examination?	Yes ____	No__
If yes, was it in the past 3 months?	Yes ____	No__
less than 1 year? Yes ____ No ____, 1-2 years?	Yes ____	No__
over 2 years? Yes ____ No ____, Never?	Yes ____	No__
Have you ever had an abnormal prostate examination?	Yes ____	No__
If yes, when? ____/____/____		
Have you ever had a vasectomy?	Yes ____	No__
If yes, when? ____/____/____ Age at time? ____		

Have you recently been experiencing any of the following:

Symptom	Yes	No	When occurred	Currently
Shortness of breath:	____	____	_____	_____
Excessive coughing:	____	____	_____	_____
Coughed up blood:	____	____	_____	_____
Coughed up sputum:	____	____	_____	_____
Chest pain:	____	____	_____	_____
Chest pressure:	____	____	_____	_____
Tightness in arms:	____	____	_____	_____
Excessive sweating:	____	____	_____	_____
Nausea:	____	____	_____	_____
Heart pounding:	____	____	_____	_____
Blurred vision:	____	____	_____	_____
Double vision:	____	____	_____	_____
Leg or foot swelling:	____	____	_____	_____
Dizziness:	____	____	_____	_____
Weakness:	____	____	_____	_____
Numbness:	____	____	_____	_____
Incontinence:	____	____	_____	_____
Excessive Thirst:	____	____	_____	_____
Depression:	____	____	_____	_____

OTHER

_____	____	____	_____	_____
_____	____	____	_____	_____
_____	____	____	_____	_____

Are you at risk for AIDS or HIV?   Yes ____ No ____
Have you recently been exposed to any infectious disease?   Yes ____No____

Have you ever smoked? Yes ____ No ____ If yes, how many packs per day? __
Do you smoke now?   Yes ____ No____
If smoking, is your choice: Cigarettes ____ Cigars ____ Pipe ____ Other _____
Do you drink alcohol? Occasionally ____ Socially ____ Daily ____ Never____

What caffeine do you consume daily? Coffee ____ Tea ____ Soda Pop _____
Total 8 Oz. servings of caffeine daily?   0-2 ____   3-5 ____   6 or more ____

Do you routinely exercise?   Daily _____   2-3 days per week _____
3-5 days per week _____   Never _____

How many servings of fruit do you eat daily?   1-2 ____ 3-5 ____ None ____
How many servings of vegetables do you eat daily? 1-2 ____ 3-5 ____ None ____
How many Glasses of water do you drink daily?   1-3 ____ 4-6 ____ 7-10 ____

Have you or any blood relatives ever been diagnosed with cancer?

Type of cancer	You	Other	Treated	Year
Brain cancer	____	____	____	____
Breast cancer	____	____	____	____
Colon cancer	____	____	____	____
Leukemia	____	____	____	____
Lung cancer	____	____	____	____
Ovarian cancer	____	____	____	____
Pancreatic cancer	____	____	____	____
Prostate cancer	____	____	____	____
Rectal cancer	____	____	____	____
Thyroid cancer	____	____	____	____
OTHER				
_____	____	____	____	____
_____	____	____	____	____
_____	____	____	____	____

Quarterly Questionnaire Review

(For use in Chronic Disease and Short Term Acute Illness)

Time covered: ___/___/___ through ___/___/___

Patient's name: _____ DOB: ___/___/___
Current age: _____ Gender: Female _____ Male _____
Height ____Ft ____In Weight ____LB
Recent weight gain: Yes____ No ____ Recent weight loss: Yes____ No ____
Family doctor: _____

Has patient had new x-rays in previous three months? Yes ____ No ___
If yes, x-rays requested: _____
_____
Name of facility that performed x-rays: _____
Were there new findings from these x-rays? Yes ____ No____
New findings: _____
_____
_____
Were other tests or procedures requested in previous three months? Yes ___ No___
Name of procedures performed: _____
_____
Does patient have copy of reports from x-rays and procedures? Yes ___ No ____

Have you recently traveled outside of the United States? Yes ____No____
If yes, did this travel require specific inoculations? Yes ____No ____
If yes, what ones were required? _____
_____
Did you have any adverse reaction to the inoculations? Yes ____No ____
If yes, what type of reaction? _____
Date of reaction: ___/___/___ Was treatment needed? Yes ____No ____
Have you recently received a blood transfusion? Yes ____No ____
If yes, how many units were required? _____
Did you ever receive blood transfusions before 1980? Yes ___No ____
between 1980-1990? Yes ____ No ____, after 1990? Yes ____No ____

84

Name of **All** medications currently taking prescribed or not - including vitamins, over the counter medications (OTC), herbal or natural therapy, pain relievers, cold medication, laxatives, nutritional supplement (such as Ensure), diuretics or contraceptives:

Medication	*Supplement/Other*	*Dosage*	*How often*
_____	_____	_____	_____
_____	_____	_____	_____
_____	_____	_____	_____
_____	_____	_____	_____
_____	_____	_____	_____
_____	_____	_____	_____
_____	_____	_____	_____
_____	_____	_____	_____
_____	_____	_____	_____
_____	_____	_____	_____

To be completed by FEMALE only:

Have you had a pelvic exam with Pap smear in past 3 months? Yes ___ No ___
If not, have you had one in the past year?   Yes ___ No ___
in the past 1-3 years?   Yes ____ No ____,   3-5 years?   Yes ___ No ___
Has it been more than 5 years? Yes ____ No ____
Have you ever been informed that your Pap smear was abnormal? Yes ___ No ___
Have you had a hysterectomy? Yes ____ No ____ If yes, when? ___/___/___
Age at time? _____ Are you on hormone replacement?   Yes ___ No ___

Do you routinely have a mammogram?   Yes ___ No ___
When was your last mammogram: within the past 3 months?   Yes ___ No ___
Less than 1 year?   Yes ____ No ____,   1-2 years?   Yes ___ No ___
2-5 years?   Yes ____ No ____, Never?   Yes ____ No ____
Are your periods regular? Yes ____ No ____ Last period?   ___/___/___
Are you taking birth control pills?   Yes ___ No ___
Are you currently pregnant?   Yes ___ No ___

85

To be completed by MALE only:

Have you ever had a prostate examination?		Yes ___ No ___
If yes, was it in the past 3 months?		Yes ___ No ___
less than 1 year? Yes ____ No ____, 1-2 years?		Yes ___ No ___
over 2 years? Yes ____ No ____, Never?		Yes ___ No ___
Have you ever had an abnormal prostate examination?		Yes ___ No ___
If yes, when? ____/____/____		
Have you ever had a vasectomy?		Yes ___ No ___
If yes, when? ____/____/____ Age at time? _____		

Have you recently been experiencing any of the following:

Symptom	Yes	No	When occurred	Currently
Shortness of breath:	___	___	_____	_____
Excessive coughing:	___	___	_____	_____
Coughed up blood:	___	___	_____	_____
Coughed up sputum:	___	___	_____	_____
Chest pain:	___	___	_____	_____
Chest pressure:	___	___	_____	_____
Tightness in arms:	___	___	_____	_____
Excessive sweating:	___	___	_____	_____
Nausea:	___	___	_____	_____
Heart pounding:	___	___	_____	_____
Blurred vision:	___	___	_____	_____
Double vision:	___	___	_____	_____
Leg or foot swelling:	___	___	_____	_____
Dizziness:	___	___	_____	_____
Weakness:	___	___	_____	_____
Numbness:	___	___	_____	_____
Incontinence:	___	___	_____	_____
Excessive Thirst:	___	___	_____	_____
Depression:	___	___	_____	_____

OTHER

_____	___	___	_____	_____
_____	___	___	_____	_____
_____	___	___	_____	_____

Are you at risk for AIDS or HIV? Yes ___ No ___
Have you recently been exposed to any infectious disease? Yes ___ No ___

Have you ever smoked? Yes ___ No ___ If yes, how many packs per day? __
Do you smoke now? Yes ___ No ___
If smoking, is your choice: Cigarettes ___ Cigars ___ Pipe ___ Other ___
Do you drink alcohol? Occasionally ___ Socially ___ Daily ___ Never ___

What caffeine do you consume daily? Coffee ___ Tea ___ Soda Pop ___
Total 8 Oz. servings of caffeine daily? 0-2 ___ 3-5 ___ 6 or more ___

Do you routinely exercise? Daily ___ 2-3 days per week ___
3-5 days per week ___ Never ___

How many servings of fruit do you eat daily? 1-2 ___ 3-5 ___ None ___
How many servings of vegetables do you eat daily? 1-2 ___ 3-5 ___ None ___
How many Glasses of water do you drink daily? 1-3 ___ 4-6 ___ 7-10 ___

Have you or any blood relatives ever been diagnosed with cancer?

Type of cancer	You	Other	Treated	Year
Brain cancer	___	___	___	___
Breast cancer	___	___	___	___
Colon cancer	___	___	___	___
Leukemia	___	___	___	___
Lung cancer	___	___	___	___
Ovarian cancer	___	___	___	___
Pancreatic cancer	___	___	___	___
Prostate cancer	___	___	___	___
Rectal cancer	___	___	___	___
Thyroid cancer	___	___	___	___
OTHER				
_____	___	___	___	___
_____	___	___	___	___
_____	___	___	___	___

87

Quarterly Questionnaire Review

(For use in Chronic Disease and Short Term Acute Illness)

Time covered: ___/___/___ through ___/___/___

Patient's name: _____ DOB: ___/___/____
Current age: _____ Gender: Female _____ Male _____
Height ____Ft ____In   Weight ____LB
Recent weight gain: Yes____ No ____   Recent weight loss: Yes____ No ____
Family doctor: _____

Has patient had new x-rays in previous three months?   Yes ____ No ___
If yes, x-rays requested: _____
_____

Name of facility that performed x-rays: _____
Were there new findings from these x-rays?   Yes ____ No____
New findings: _____
_____
_____

Were other tests or procedures requested in previous three months? Yes ___ No___
Name of procedures performed: _____

Does patient have copy of reports from x-rays and procedures? Yes ___ No ____

Have you recently traveled outside of the United States?   Yes ____No____
If yes, did this travel require specific inoculations?   Yes ____No ____
If yes, what ones were required? _____

Did you have any adverse reaction to the inoculations?   Yes ____No ____
If yes, what type of reaction? _____
Date of reaction: ____/___/____ Was treatment needed? Yes ____ No ____
Have you recently received a blood transfusion?   Yes ____No ____
If yes, how many units were required? _____
Did you ever receive blood transfusions before 1980?   Yes ____No ____
between 1980-1990? Yes ____ No ____, after 1990?   Yes ____No ____

Name of **All** medications currently taking prescribed or not - including vitamins, over the counter medications (OTC), herbal or natural therapy, pain relievers, cold medication, laxatives, nutritional supplement (such as Ensure), diuretics or contraceptives:

Medication	_Supplement/Other_	_Dosage_	_How often_
_____	_____	_____	_____
_____	_____	_____	_____
_____	_____	_____	_____
_____	_____	_____	_____
_____	_____	_____	_____
_____	_____	_____	_____
_____	_____	_____	_____
_____	_____	_____	_____
_____	_____	_____	_____
_____	_____	_____	_____
_____	_____	_____	_____

To be completed by FEMALE only:

Have you had a pelvic exam with Pap smear in past 3 months? Yes ___ No ___
If not, have you had one in the past year? Yes ___ No ___
in the past 1-3 years? Yes ___ No ___, 3-5 years? Yes ___ No ___
Has it been more than 5 years? Yes ___ No ___
Have you ever been informed that your Pap smear was abnormal? Yes ___ No ___
Have you had a hysterectomy? Yes ___ No ___ If yes, when? ___/___/___
Age at time? ___ Are you on hormone replacement? Yes ___ No ___

Do you routinely have a mammogram? Yes ___ No ___
When was your last mammogram: within the past 3 months? Yes ___ No ___
Less than 1 year? Yes ___ No ___, 1-2 years? Yes ___ No ___
2-5 years? Yes ___ No ___, Never? Yes ___ No ___
Are your periods regular? Yes ___ No ___ Last period? ___/___/___
Are you taking birth control pills? Yes ___ No ___
Are you currently pregnant? Yes ___ No ___

To be completed by MALE only:

Have you ever had a prostate examination?	Yes ___ No ___
If yes, was it in the past 3 months?	Yes ___ No ___
less than 1 year? Yes ____ No ____, 1-2 years?	Yes ___ No ___
over 2 years? Yes ____ No ____, Never?	Yes ___ No ___
Have you ever had an abnormal prostate examination?	Yes ___ No ___
If yes, when? ___/___/___	
Have you ever had a vasectomy?	Yes ___ No ___
If yes, when? ___/___/___ Age at time? _____	

Have you recently been experiencing any of the following:

Symptom	Yes	No	When occurred	Currently
Shortness of breath:	____	____	_____	_____
Excessive coughing:	____	____	_____	_____
Coughed up blood:	____	____	_____	_____
Coughed up sputum:	____	____	_____	_____
Chest pain:	____	____	_____	_____
Chest pressure:	____	____	_____	_____
Tightness in arms:	____	____	_____	_____
Excessive sweating	____	____	_____	_____
Nausea:	____	____	_____	_____
Heart pounding:	____	____	_____	_____
Blurred vision:	____	____	_____	_____
Double vision:	____	____	_____	_____
Leg or foot swelling:	____	____	_____	_____
Dizziness:	____	____	_____	_____
Weakness:	____	____	_____	_____
Numbness:	____	____	_____	_____
Incontinence:	____	____	_____	_____
Excessive Thirst:	____	____	_____	_____
Depression:	____	____	_____	_____
OTHER				
_____	____	____	_____	_____
_____	____	____	_____	_____
_____	____	____	_____	_____

Are you at risk for AIDS or HIV?   Yes ___ No ___
Have you recently been exposed to any infectious disease?   Yes ___ No ___

Have you ever smoked? Yes ___ No ___ If yes, how many packs per day? __
Do you smoke now?   Yes ___ No ___
If smoking, is your choice: Cigarettes ___ Cigars ___ Pipe ___ Other ___
Do you drink alcohol? Occasionally ___ Socially ___ Daily ___ Never ___

What caffeine do you consume daily?   Coffee ___   Tea ___   Soda Pop ___
Total 8 Oz. servings of caffeine daily?   0-2 ___   3-5 ___   6 or more ___

Do you routinely exercise?   Daily ___   2-3 days per week ___
3-5 days per week ___   Never ___

How many servings of fruit do you eat daily?   1-2 ___ 3-5 ___ None ___
How many servings of vegetables do you eat daily? 1-2 ___ 3-5 ___ None ___
How many Glasses of water do you drink daily?   1-3 ___ 4-6 ___ 7-10 ___

Have you or any blood relatives ever been diagnosed with cancer?

Type of cancer	You	Other	Treated	Year
Brain cancer	___	___	___	___
Breast cancer	___	___	___	___
Colon cancer	___	___	___	___
Leukemia	___	___	___	___
Lung cancer	___	___	___	___
Ovarian cancer	___	___	___	___
Pancreatic cancer	___	___	___	___
Prostate cancer	___	___	___	___
Rectal cancer	___	___	___	___
Thyroid cancer	___	___	___	___
OTHER				
_____	___	___	___	___
_____	___	___	___	___
_____	___	___	___	___

ADMISSIONS

"As a man thinketh in his heart, so he is." Proverbs 23:7

Admission
To
Hospital, Rehab Center or Long Term Facility

Date of admission ___/___/___ Time of admission ___:___ AM/PM

Patient name: _____

Name of facility:_____

Doctor admitting: _____

Admitting diagnosis: _____

Transported to facility by: _____

Condition at admission: Conscious: Yes ____   No ____

Vitals: Temperature _____   Blood Pressure ___/___   Pulse ____

High fever: Yes ____   No ____ Bleeding: Yes ____   No ____

Short of breath: Yes ____   No ____ Chest Pain: Yes ____   No ____

Injury related: Yes ____   No ____ Fractures: Yes ____   No ____

Surgery needed: Yes ____   No ____ If yes, type of surgery _____

Other:_____

Special Instructions:_____

_____

Dietary Restrictions:_____

Room Assignment: Semi-Private: Yes ____   No ____

Private: Yes ____   No ____   Intensive Care: Yes ____   No ____

Room Number and bed: _____-_____ Special bed required: Yes ____ No ____

New Prescriptions, Old Prescriptions, dosage, time to take and reason to start or stop specific prescription:

Prescription	New	Old	Dosage	Time	Reason
_____	____	____	_____	_____	____
_____	____	____	_____	_____	____
_____	____	____	_____	_____	____
_____	____	____	_____	_____	____

Doctor consultations requested:

Doctor   Specialty

_____   _____
_____   _____
_____   _____
_____   _____

Admission Summary

(As described by patient, parent, guardian or family member)
***
(Be sure to compare with official admission summary from facility, request corrections as needed and obtain a copy of correction)

_____
_____
_____
_____
_____
_____
_____
_____
_____
_____
_____
_____
_____
_____
_____

Admission
To
Hospital, Rehab Center or Long Term Facility

Date of admission ___/___/___ Time of admission ____:____ AM/PM
Patient name: _____
Name of facility: _____
Doctor admitting: _____
Admitting diagnosis: _____
Transported to facility by: _____
Condition at admission: Conscious: Yes ____   No ____
Vitals: Temperature _____   Blood Pressure ____/____   Pulse _____
High fever: Yes ____ No ____ Bleeding: Yes ____ No ____
Short of breath: Yes ____ No ____ Chest Pain: Yes ____ No ____
Injury related: Yes ____ No ____ Fractures: Yes ____ No ____
Surgery needed: Yes ____ No ____ If yes, type of surgery _____
Other:_____

SpecialInstructions:_____
_____

Dietary Restrictions: _____

Room Assignment: Semi-Private: Yes ____   No ____
Private: Yes ____   No ____   Intensive Care: Yes ____   No ____
Room Number and bed: _____-_____ Special bed required: Yes ____ No ____

New Prescriptions, Old Prescriptions, dosage, time to take and reason to
start or stop specific prescription:

Prescription	New	Old	Dosage	Time	Reason
_____	___	___	_____	_____	____
_____	___	___	_____	_____	____
_____	___	___	_____	_____	____
_____	___	___	_____	_____	____

Doctor consultations requested:

Doctor   Specialty

_____   _____
_____   _____
_____   _____
_____   _____

Admission Summary

(As described by patient, parent, guardian or family member)
***
(Be sure to compare with official admission summary from facility,   request
corrections as needed and obtain a copy of correction)

_____
_____
_____
_____
_____
_____
_____
_____
_____
_____
_____
_____
_____
_____
_____
_____

Admission
To
Hospital, Rehab Center or Long Term Facility

Date of admission ___/___/___ Time of admission ___:___ AM/PM
Patient name: _____
Name of facility: _____
Doctor admitting: _____
Admitting diagnosis: _____
Transported to facility by: _____
Condition at admission: Conscious: Yes ____   No ____
Vitals: Temperature ____   Blood Pressure ___/___   Pulse ____
High fever: Yes ____ No ____ Bleeding: Yes ____ No ____
Short of breath: Yes ____ No ____ Chest Pain: Yes ____ No ____
Injury related: Yes ____ No ____ Fractures: Yes ____ No ____
Surgery needed: Yes ____ No ____ If yes, type of surgery _____
Other:_____

SpecialInstructions:_____
_____

Dietary Restrictions: _____

Room Assignment: Semi-Private: Yes ____   No ____
Private: Yes ____   No ____   Intensive Care: Yes ____ No ____
Room Number and bed: ____-____ Special bed required: Yes ____ No ____

New Prescriptions, Old Prescriptions, dosage, time to take and reason to start or stop specific prescription:

Prescription	New	Old	Dosage	Time	Reason
_____	____	____	_____	_____	____
_____	____	____	_____	_____	____
_____	____	____	_____	_____	____
_____	____	____	_____	_____	____

Doctor consultations requested:

Doctor   Specialty

_____   _____
_____   _____
_____   _____
_____   _____

Admission Summary

(As described by patient, parent, guardian or family member)
***
(Be sure to compare with official admission summary from facility, request corrections as needed and obtain a copy of correction)

_____
_____
_____
_____
_____
_____
_____
_____
_____
_____
_____
_____
_____
_____
_____
_____
_____

Admission
To
Hospital, Rehab Center or Long Term Facility

Date of admission ___/___/___ Time of admission ___:___ AM/PM

Patient name: _____

Name of facility: _____

Doctor admitting: _____

Admitting diagnosis: _____

Transported to facility by: _____

Condition at admission: Conscious: Yes ____   No ____

Vitals: Temperature ____   Blood Pressure ___/___   Pulse ____

High fever: Yes ____ No ____ Bleeding: Yes ____ No ____

Short of breath: Yes ____ No ____ Chest Pain: Yes ____ No ____

Injury related: Yes ____ No ____ Fractures: Yes ____ No ____

Surgery needed: Yes ____ No ____ If yes, type of surgery _____

Other:_____

SpecialInstructions:_____

_____

Dietary Restrictions: _____

Room Assignment: Semi-Private: Yes ____   No ____

Private: Yes ____   No ____   Intensive Care: Yes ____ No ____

Room Number and bed: ____-____ Special bed required: Yes ____ No ____

New Prescriptions, Old Prescriptions, dosage, time to take and reason to start or stop specific prescription;

Prescription	New	Old	Dosage	Time	Reason
_____	____	____	_____	_____	____
_____	____	____	_____	_____	____
_____	____	____	_____	_____	____
_____	____	____	_____	_____	____

Doctor consultations requested:

Doctor   Specialty

_____   _____
_____   _____
_____   _____
_____   _____

Admission Summary

(As described by patient, parent, guardian or family member)
***
(Be sure to compare with official admission summary from facility,   request corrections as needed and obtain a copy of correction)

_____
_____
_____
_____
_____
_____
_____
_____
_____
_____
_____
_____
_____
_____
_____
_____

DISCHARGES

"A friend loves at all times."　　　　*Proverbs 17:17*

Discharge From:
Hospital, Rehab Center or Long Term Facility

Date of discharge ___/___/___ Time of discharge ____:____ AM/PM
Patient name: _____
Name of facility: _____
Doctor discharging: _____
Discharge diagnosis: _____
Transported home by: _____

New Instruction: _____
_____
_____

Restrictions: _____
_____

Dietary changes: _____
_____

New Prescriptions, Old Prescriptions, dosage, time to take and reason to start or stop specific prescription:

Prescription	*New*	*Old*	*Dosage*	*Time*	*Reason*
_____	___	___	_____	_____	___
_____	___	___	_____	_____	___
_____	___	___	_____	_____	___
_____	___	___	_____	_____	___

Follow up appointments scheduled: Yes _____   No _____
Time of next appointment: Day_____ Time ____:____ AM/PM
Location of next appointment: _____

Special In-Home care or treatments needed: Yes _____   No _____
Special equipment needed (such as oxygen)   Yes _____   No _____
Name of provider: _____
Providers Phone No. ( )_____-_____

100

Discharge Summary

(As described by patient, parent, guardian or family member)
***
(Be sure to compare with official discharge summary from facility, request corrections as needed and obtain a copy of correction)

_____
_____
_____
_____
_____
_____
_____
_____
_____
_____
_____
_____

Name(s) of doctor you've requested a summary to be sent to:

Name: _____ Specialty: _____
Address: _____

Name: _____ Specialty: _____
Address: _____

Name: _____ Specialty: _____
Address: _____

Name: _____ Specialty: _____
Address: _____

Discharge From:
Hospital, Rehab Center or Long Term Facility

Date of discharge ___/___/___ Time of discharge ____:____ AM/PM
Patient name: _____
Name of facility: _____
Doctor discharging: _____
Discharge diagnosis: _____
Transported home by: _____

New Instruction: _____
_____
_____

Restrictions: _____
_____

Dietary changes: _____
_____

New Prescriptions, Old Prescriptions, dosage, time to take and reason to start or stop specific prescription:

Prescription	New	Old	Dosage	Time	Reason
_____	___	___	_____	_____	_____
_____	___	___	_____	_____	_____
_____	___	___	_____	_____	_____
_____	___	___	_____	_____	_____

Follow up appointments scheduled: Yes _____ No _____
Time of next appointment: Day_____ Time ____:____AM/PM
Location of next appointment: _____

Special In-Home care or treatments needed: Yes _____ No _____
Special equipment needed (such as oxygen) Yes _____ No _____
Name of provider: _____
Providers Phone No. ( )_____-_____

102

Discharge Summary

(As described by patient, parent, guardian or family member)
***
(Be sure to compare with official discharge summary from facility, request corrections as needed and obtain a copy of correction)

_____
_____
_____
_____
_____
_____
_____
_____
_____
_____
_____
_____

<u>Name(s) of doctor you've requested a summary to be sent to:</u>

Name: _____   Specialty:_____
Address: _____

Name: _____   Specialty:_____
Address: _____

Name: _____   Specialty:_____
Address: _____

Name: _____   Specialty:_____
Address: _____

Discharge From:
Hospital, Rehab Center or Long Term Facility

Date of discharge ___/___/___ Time of discharge ____:____ AM/PM
Patient name: _____
Name of facility: _____
Doctor discharging: _____
Discharge diagnosis: _____
Transported home by: _____

New Instruction: _____
_____
_____

Restrictions: _____
_____

Dietary changes: _____
_____

New Prescriptions, Old Prescriptions, dosage, time to take and reason to start or stop specific prescription:

Prescription	New	Old	Dosage	Time	Reason
_____	___	___	_____	_____	_____
_____	___	___	_____	_____	_____
_____	___	___	_____	_____	_____
_____	___	___	_____	_____	_____

Follow up appointments scheduled: Yes _____ No _____
Time of next appointment: Day_____ Time ____:____AM/PM
Location of next appointment: _____

Special In-Home care or treatments needed: Yes _____ No _____
Special equipment needed (such as oxygen) Yes _____ No _____
Name of provider: _____
Providers Phone No. (   )_____-_____

Discharge Summary

(As described by patient, parent, guardian or family member)
***
(Be sure to compare with official discharge summary from facility, request corrections as needed and obtain a copy of correction)

_____
_____
_____
_____
_____
_____
_____
_____
_____
_____
_____

Name(s) of doctor you've requested a summary to be sent to:

Name: _____ Specialty: _____
Address: _____

Name: _____ Specialty: _____
Address: _____

Name: _____ Specialty: _____
Address: _____

Name: _____ Specialty: _____
Address: _____

Discharge From:
Hospital, Rehab Center or Long Term Facility

Date of discharge ___/___/___ Time of discharge ____:____ AM/PM
Patient name: _____
Name of facility: _____
Doctor discharging: _____
Discharge diagnosis: _____
Transported home by: _____

New Instruction: _____
_____
_____

Restrictions: _____
_____

Dietary changes: _____
_____

New Prescriptions, Old Prescriptions, dosage, time to take and reason to start or stop specific prescription:

Prescription	*New*	*Old*	*Dosage*	*Time*	*Reason*
_____	___	___	_____	_____	___
_____	___	___	_____	_____	___
_____	___	___	_____	_____	___
_____	___	___	_____	_____	___

Follow up appointments scheduled: Yes _____   No _____
Time of next appointment: Day_____ Time ____:____ AM/PM
Location of next appointment: _____

Special In-Home care or treatments needed: Yes _____   No _____
Special equipment needed (such as oxygen)   Yes _____   No _____
Name of provider: _____
Providers Phone No. (   )_____-_____

106

Discharge Summary

(As described by patient, parent, guardian or family member)
***
(Be sure to compare with official discharge summary from facility, request corrections as needed and obtain a copy of correction)

_____
_____
_____
_____
_____
_____
_____
_____
_____
_____
_____
_____

Name(s) of doctor you've requested a summary to be sent to:

Name: _____ Specialty: _____
Address: _____

Name: _____ Specialty: _____
Address: _____

Name: _____ Specialty: _____
Address: _____

Name: _____ Specialty: _____
Address: _____

_____

MORE

JOURNAL

PAGES

"Instruct a wise man and he will be wiser still; teach a righteous man and he will add to his learning." Proverbs 9:9

Journal Notes

Journal Notes

Journal Notes

Journal Notes

Journal Notes

Journal Notes

Journal Notes

_____
_____
_____
_____
_____
_____
_____
_____
_____
_____
_____
_____
_____
_____
_____
_____
_____
_____
_____
_____
_____
_____
_____
_____
_____
_____
_____
_____

Journal Notes

Journal Notes

Journal Notes

Journal Notes

Journal Notes

MORE

EXPENDITURES

"He who heeds discipline shows the way to life, but whoever ignores correction leads others astray." **Proverbs 10:17**

Expenditures: Parking/Food/Phone Calls/Miscellaneous

Sunday   Date___/___/___
A. Breakfast_____ Amount$____.____   Comments_____
B. Lunch _____ Amount$____.____   Comments_____
C. Dinner _____ Amount$____.____   Comments_____
D. Parking _____ Amount$____.____   Comments_____
E. Phone _____ Amount$____.____   Comments_____
F. Misc. _____ Amount$____.____   Comments_____

Monday   Date___/___/___
A. Breakfast_____ Amount$____.____   Comments_____
B. Lunch _____ Amount$____.____   Comments_____
C. Dinner _____ Amount$____.____   Comments_____
D. Parking _____ Amount$____.____   Comments_____
E. Phone _____ Amount$____.____   Comments_____
F. Misc. _____ Amount$____.____   Comments_____

Tuesday   Date___/___/___
A. Breakfast_____ Amount$____.____   Comments_____
B. Lunch _____ Amount$____.____   Comments_____
C. Dinner _____ Amount$____.____   Comments_____
D. Parking _____ Amount$____.____   Comments_____
E. Phone _____ Amount$____.____   Comments_____
F. Misc. _____ Amount$____.____   Comments_____

Wednesday   Date___/___/___
A. Breakfast_____ Amount$____.____   Comments_____
B. Lunch _____ Amount$____.____   Comments_____
C. Dinner _____ Amount$____.____   Comments_____
D. Parking _____ Amount$____.____   Comments_____
E. Phone _____ Amount$____.____   Comments_____
F. Misc. _____ Amount$____.____   Comments_____

Expenditures: Parking/Food/Phone Calls/Miscellaneous

Thursday   Date___/___/___
A. Breakfast_____ Amount$____.____   Comments_____
B. Lunch   _____ Amount$____.____   Comments_____
C. Dinner   _____ Amount$____.____   Comments_____
D. Parking   _____ Amount$____.____   Comments_____
E. Phone   _____ Amount$____.____   Comments_____
F. Misc.   _____ Amount$____.____   Comments_____

Friday   Date___/___/___
A. Breakfast_____ Amount$____.____   Comments_____
B. Lunch   _____ Amount$____.____   Comments_____
C. Dinner   _____ Amount$____.____   Comments_____
D. Parking   _____ Amount$____.____   Comments_____
E. Phone   _____ Amount$____.____   Comments_____
F. Misc.   _____ Amount$____.____   Comments_____

Saturday   Date___/___/___
A. Breakfast_____ Amount$____.____   Comments_____
B. Lunch   _____ Amount$____.____   Comments_____
C. Dinner   _____ Amount$____.____   Comments_____
D. Parking   _____ Amount$____.____   Comments_____
E. Phone   _____ Amount$____.____   Comments_____
F. Misc.   _____ Amount$____.____   Comments_____

Additional Comments _____
_____
_____
_____
_____
_____

121

Expenditures: Parking/Food/Phone Calls/Miscellaneous

Sunday   Date____/____/____
A. Breakfast_____ Amount$____.____   Comments_____
B. Lunch _____ Amount$____.____   Comments_____
C. Dinner _____ Amount$____.____   Comments_____
D. Parking _____ Amount$____.____   Comments_____
E. Phone _____ Amount$____.____   Comments_____
F. Misc. _____ Amount$____.____   Comments_____

Monday   Date____/____/____
A. Breakfast_____ Amount$____.____   Comments_____
B. Lunch _____ Amount$____.____   Comments_____
C. Dinner _____ Amount$____.____   Comments_____
D. Parking _____ Amount$____.____   Comments_____
E. Phone _____ Amount$____.____   Comments_____
F. Misc. _____ Amount$____.____   Comments_____

Tuesday   Date____/____/____
A. Breakfast_____ Amount$____.____   Comments_____
B. Lunch _____ Amount$____.____   Comments_____
C. Dinner _____ Amount$____.____   Comments_____
D. Parking _____ Amount$____.____   Comments_____
E. Phone _____ Amount$____.____   Comments_____
F. Misc. _____ Amount$____.____   Comments_____

Wednesday   Date____/____/____
A. Breakfast_____ Amount$____.____   Comments_____
B. Lunch _____ Amount$____.____   Comments_____
C. Dinner _____ Amount$____.____   Comments_____
D. Parking _____ Amount$____.____   Comments_____
E. Phone _____ Amount$____.____   Comments_____
F. Misc. _____ Amount$____.____   Comments_____

Expenditures: Parking/Food/Phone Calls/Miscellaneous

Thursday   Date___/___/___
A. Breakfast_____ Amount$___.___   Comments_____
B. Lunch   _____ Amount$___.___   Comments_____
C. Dinner   _____ Amount$___.___   Comments_____
D. Parking _____ Amount$___.___   Comments_____
E. Phone   _____ Amount$___.___   Comments_____
F. Misc.   _____ Amount$___.___   Comments_____

Friday   Date___/___/___
A. Breakfast_____ Amount$___.___   Comments_____
B. Lunch   _____ Amount$___.___   Comments_____
C. Dinner   _____ Amount$___.___   Comments_____
D. Parking _____ Amount$___.___   Comments_____
E. Phone   _____ Amount$___.___   Comments_____
F. Misc.   _____ Amount$___.___   Comments_____

Saturday   Date___/___/___
A. Breakfast_____ Amount$___.___   Comments_____
B. Lunch   _____ Amount$___.___   Comments_____
C. Dinner   _____ Amount$___.___   Comments_____
D. Parking _____ Amount$___.___   Comments_____
E. Phone   _____ Amount$___.___   Comments_____
F. Misc.   _____ Amount$___.___   Comments_____

Additional Comments _____
_____
_____
_____
_____
_____

Expenditures: Parking/Food/Phone Calls/Miscellaneous

Sunday   Date___/___/___
A. Breakfast_____ Amount$____.____   Comments_____
B. Lunch   _____ Amount$____.____   Comments_____
C. Dinner   _____ Amount$____.____   Comments_____
D. Parking _____ Amount$____.____   Comments_____
E. Phone   _____ Amount$____.____   Comments_____
F. Misc.   _____ Amount$____.____   Comments_____

Monday   Date___/___/___
A. Breakfast_____ Amount$____.____   Comments_____
B. Lunch   _____ Amount$____.____   Comments_____
C. Dinner   _____ Amount$____.____   Comments_____
D. Parking _____ Amount$____.____   Comments_____
E. Phone   _____ Amount$____.____   Comments_____
F. Misc.   _____ Amount$____.____   Comments_____

Tuesday   Date___/___/___
A. Breakfast_____ Amount$____.____   Comments_____
B. Lunch   _____ Amount$____.____   Comments_____
C. Dinner   _____ Amount$____.____   Comments_____
D. Parking _____ Amount$____.____   Comments_____
E. Phone   _____ Amount$____.____   Comments_____
F. Misc.   _____ Amount$____.____   Comments_____

Wednesday   Date___/___/___
A. Breakfast_____ Amount$____.____   Comments_____
B. Lunch   _____ Amount$____.____   Comments_____
C. Dinner   _____ Amount$____.____   Comments_____
D. Parking _____ Amount$____.____   Comments_____
E. Phone   _____ Amount$____.____   Comments_____
F. Misc.   _____ Amount$____.____   Comments_____

Expenditures: Parking/Food/Phone Calls/Miscellaneous

Thursday   Date___/___/___
A. Breakfast_____ Amount$____.____   Comments_____
B. Lunch _____ Amount$____.____   Comments_____
C. Dinner _____ Amount$____.____   Comments_____
D. Parking _____ Amount$____.____   Comments_____
E. Phone _____ Amount$____.____   Comments_____
F. Misc. _____ Amount$____.____   Comments_____

Friday   Date___/___/___
A. Breakfast_____ Amount$____.____   Comments_____
B. Lunch _____ Amount$____.____   Comments_____
C. Dinner _____ Amount$____.____   Comments_____
D. Parking _____ Amount$____.____   Comments_____
E. Phone _____ Amount$____.____   Comments_____
F. Misc. _____ Amount$____.____   Comments_____

Saturday   Date___/___/___
A. Breakfast_____ Amount$____.____   Comments_____
B. Lunch _____ Amount$____.____   Comments_____
C. Dinner _____ Amount$____.____   Comments_____
D. Parking _____ Amount$____.____   Comments_____
E. Phone _____ Amount$____.____   Comments_____
F. Misc. _____ Amount$____.____   Comments_____

Additional Comments _____
_____
_____
_____
_____
_____

Expenditures: Parking/Food/Phone Calls/Miscellaneous

Sunday   Date___/___/___
A. Breakfast_____ Amount$___.___   Comments_____
B. Lunch   _____ Amount$___.___   Comments_____
C. Dinner   _____ Amount$___.___   Comments_____
D. Parking _____ Amount$___.___   Comments_____
E. Phone   _____ Amount$___.___   Comments_____
F. Misc.   _____ Amount$___.___   Comments_____

Monday   Date___/___/___
A. Breakfast_____ Amount$___.___   Comments_____
B. Lunch   _____ Amount$___.___   Comments_____
C. Dinner   _____ Amount$___.___   Comments_____
D. Parking _____ Amount$___.___   Comments_____
E. Phone   _____ Amount$___.___   Comments_____
F. Misc.   _____ Amount$___.___   Comments_____

Tuesday   Date___/___/___
A. Breakfast_____ Amount$___.___   Comments_____
B. Lunch   _____ Amount$___.___   Comments_____
C. Dinner   _____ Amount$___.___   Comments_____
D. Parking _____ Amount$___.___   Comments_____
E. Phone   _____ Amount$___.___   Comments_____
F. Misc.   _____ Amount$___.___   Comments_____

Wednesday   Date___/___/___
A. Breakfast_____ Amount$___.___   Comments_____
B. Lunch   _____ Amount$___.___   Comments_____
C. Dinner   _____ Amount$___.___   Comments_____
D. Parking _____ Amount$___.___   Comments_____
E. Phone   _____ Amount$___.___   Comments_____
F. Misc.   _____ Amount$___.___   Comments_____

Expenditures: Parking/Food/Phone Calls/Miscellaneous

Thursday   Date___/___/___
A. Breakfast_____ Amount$___.___   Comments_____
B. Lunch   _____ Amount$___.___   Comments_____
C. Dinner   _____ Amount$___.___   Comments_____
D. Parking _____ Amount$___.___   Comments_____
E. Phone   _____ Amount$___.___   Comments_____
F. Misc.   _____ Amount$___.___   Comments_____

Friday   Date___/___/___
A. Breakfast_____ Amount$___.___   Comments_____
B. Lunch   _____ Amount$___.___   Comments_____
C. Dinner   _____ Amount$___.___   Comments_____
D. Parking _____ Amount$___.___   Comments_____
E. Phone   _____ Amount$___.___   Comments_____
F. Misc.   _____ Amount$___.___   Comments_____

Saturday   Date___/___/___
A. Breakfast_____ Amount$___.___   Comments_____
B. Lunch   _____ Amount$___.___   Comments_____
C. Dinner   _____ Amount$___.___   Comments_____
D. Parking _____ Amount$___.___   Comments_____
E. Phone   _____ Amount$___.___   Comments_____
F. Misc.   _____ Amount$___.___   Comments_____

Additional Comments _____

_____
_____
_____
_____
_____

MORE

ACTIVITY

WEEKS

"A man's spirit sustains him in sickness, but a crushed spirit who can bear?"   *Proverbs 18:14*

Activity	Sun _/_/_	Mon _/_/_	Tues _/_/_
Doctors in today and what time			
Tests ordered and why?			
Previous test results			
New Medicines added			
Why new medicines?			
Old Medicines deleted			
Why Medicines deleted?			
Tests performed or Therapy			
Visitors, who and when?			

Additional Comments:

_/_/_
_/_/_
_/_/_

| Wed | Thurs | Fri | Sat |
_/_/_	_/_/_	_/_/_	_/_/_

Additional Comments:

_/_/_

_/_/_

_/_/_

Activity	Sun _/_/_	Mon _/_/_	Tues _/_/_
Doctors in today and what time			
Tests ordered and why?			
Previous test results			
New Medicines added			
Why new medicines?			
Old Medicines deleted			
Why Medicines deleted?			
Tests performed or Therapy			
Visitors, who and when?			—

Additional Comments:

_/_/_
_/_/_
_/_/_

Wed _/_/_	Thurs _/_/_	Fri _/_/_	Sat _/_/_

Additional Comments:

_/_/_
_/_/_
_/_/_

Activity	Sun ___/___/___	Mon ___/___/___	Tues ___/___/___
Doctors in today and what time			
Tests ordered and why?			
Previous test results			
New Medicines added			
Why new medicines?			
Old Medicines deleted			
Why Medicines deleted?			
Tests performed or Therapy			
Visitors, who and when?			

Additional Comments:

___/___/___ _____
___/___/___ _____
___/___/___ _____

132

Wed _/_/_	Thurs _/_/_	Fri _/_/_	Sat _/_/.

Additional Comments:

_/_/_
_/_/_
_/_/_

Activity	Sun __/__/__	Mon __/__/__	Tues __/__/__
Doctors in today and what time			
Tests ordered and why?			
Previous test results			
New Medicines added			
Why new medicines?			
Old Medicines deleted			
Why Medicines deleted?			
Tests performed or Therapy			
Visitors, who and when?			

Additional Comments:

__/__/__ _____

__/__/__ _____

__/__/__ _____

Wed _/_/_	Thurs _/_/_	Fri _/_/_	Sat _/_/_

Additional Comments:

_/_/_

_/_/_

_/_/_

MORE

NURSING

WEEKS

"He who gets wisdom loves his own soul; he who cherishes understanding prospers."   ***Proverbs 19:8***

NURSING	7AM-3PM	3PM-11PM	11PM-7AM
SUNDAY DATE / /	T_ BP_/__	T_ BP_/__	T__ BP_/__
MONDAY DATE / /	T__ BP_/__	T__ BP_/__	T__ BP_/__
TUESDAY DATE / /	T__ BP_/__	T__ BP_/__	T__ BP_/__
WEDNESDAY DATE / /	T__ BP_/__	T__ BP_/__	T__ BP_/__
THURSDAY DATE / /	T__ BP_/__	T__ BP_/__	T__ BP_/__
FRIDAY DATE / /	T__ BP_/__	T__ BP_/__	T__ BP_/__
SATURDAY DATE / /	T__ BP_/__	T__ BP_/__	T__ BP_/__

NURSING	7AM-3PM	3PM-11PM	11PM-7AM
SUNDAY DATE / /	T_BP_/_	T_BP_/_	T__BP_/_
MONDAY DATE / /	T__BP_/_	T__BP_/_	T__BP_/_
TUESDAY DATE / /	T__BP_/_	T__BP_/_	T__BP_/_
WEDNESDAY DATE / /	T__BP_/_	T__BP_/_	T__BP_/_
THURSDAY DATE / /	T__BP_/_	T__BP_/_	T__BP_/_
FRIDAY DATE / /	T__BP_/_	T__BP_/_	T__BP_/_
SATURDAY DATE / /	T__BP_/_	T__BP_/_	T__BP_/_

NURSING	7AM-3PM	3PM-11PM	11PM-7AM
SUNDAY DATE / /	T_ BP_/__	T_ BP_/_	T__ BP_/__
MONDAY DATE / /	T__ BP_/__	T__ BP_/__	T__ BP_/__
TUESDAY DATE / /	T__ BP_/__	T__ BP_/__	T__ BP_/__
WEDNESDAY DATE / /	T__ BP_/__	T__ BP_/__	T__ BP_/__
THURSDAY DATE / /	T__ BP_/__	T__ BP_/__	T__ BP_/__
FRIDAY DATE / /	T__ BP_/__	T__ BP_/__	T__ BP_/__
SATURDAY DATE / /	T__ BP_/__	T__ BP_/__	T__ BP_/__

NURSING	*7AM-3PM*	*3PM-11PM*	*11PM-7AM*
SUNDAY____ DATE _/_/__	T__BP__/__	T__BP__/__	T___BP__/__
MONDAY____ DATE _/_/__	T___BP__/__	T___BP__/__	T___BP__/__
TUESDAY____ DATE _/_/__	T___BP__/__	T___BP__/__	T___BP__/__
WEDNESDAY__ DATE _/_/__	T___BP__/__	T___BP__/__	T___BP__/__
THURSDAY____ DATE _/_/__	T___BP__/__	T___BP__/__	T___BP__/__
FRIDAY____ DATE _/_/__	T___BP__/__	T___BP__/__	T___BP__/__
SATURDAY____ DATE _/_/__	T___BP__/__	T___BP__/__	T___BP__/__

MORE

QUESTIONS:

ASK & ANSWER

"Wisdom is supreme; therefore get wisdom. Though it cost all you have, get understanding."   **Proverbs 4:7**

Questions: Asked and Answered

Date   Doctor
__ / __ / __ _____
Question: _____
_____
_____
_____

Answer: _____
_____
_____
_____

Date   Doctor
__ / __ / __ _____
Question: _____
_____
_____
_____

Answer: _____
_____
_____
_____

Date   Doctor
__ / __ / __ _____
Question: _____
_____
_____
_____

Answer: _____
_____
_____
_____

Date   Doctor
__ / __ / __ _____
Question: _____
_____
_____
_____

Answer: _____
_____
_____
_____

Date   Doctor
__ / __ / __ _____
Question: _____
_____
_____
_____

Answer: _____
_____
_____
_____

Date   Doctor
__ / __ / __ _____
Question: _____
_____
_____
_____

Answer: _____
_____
_____
_____

Questions: Asked and Answered

Date   Doctor
__/__/__   _____
Question: _____
_____
_____
_____
Answer: _____
_____
_____
_____

Date   Doctor
__/__/__   _____
Question: _____
_____
_____
_____
Answer: _____
_____
_____
_____

Date   Doctor
__/__/__   _____
Question: _____
_____
_____
_____
Answer: _____
_____
_____
_____

Date   Doctor
__/__/__   _____
Question: _____
_____
_____
_____
Answer: _____
_____
_____
_____

Date   Doctor
__/__/__   _____
Question: _____
_____
_____
_____
Answer: _____
_____
_____
_____

Date   Doctor
__/__/__   _____
Question: _____
_____
_____
_____
Answer: _____
_____
_____
_____

Questions: Asked and Answered

Date   Doctor
__/__/__   _____
Question: _____
_____
_____
_____

Answer: _____
_____
_____
_____

Date   Doctor
__/__/__   _____
Question: _____
_____
_____
_____

Answer: _____
_____
_____
_____

Date   Doctor
__/__/__   _____
Question: _____
_____
_____
_____

Answer: _____
_____
_____
_____

Date   Doctor
__/__/__   _____
Question: _____
_____
_____
_____

Answer: _____
_____
_____
_____

Date   Doctor
__/__/__   _____
Question: _____
_____
_____

Answer: _____
_____
_____
_____

Date   Doctor
__/__/__   _____
Question: _____
_____
_____

Answer: _____
_____
_____
_____

Questions: Asked and Answered

Date   Doctor   Date   Doctor
__/__/__   _____   __/__/__   _____
Question: _____   Question: _____
_____   _____
_____   _____
_____   _____
Answer: _____   Answer: _____
_____   _____
_____   _____
_____   _____

Date   Doctor   Date   Doctor
__/__/__   _____   __/__/__   _____
Question: _____   Question: _____
_____   _____
_____   _____
_____   _____
Answer: _____   Answer: _____
_____   _____
_____   _____
_____   _____

Date   Doctor   Date   Doctor
__/__/__   _____   __/__/__   _____
Question: _____   Question: _____
_____   _____
_____   _____
_____   _____
Answer: _____   Answer: _____
_____   _____
_____   _____
_____   _____

Questions: Asked and Answered

Date   Doctor
__/__/__ _____
Question: _____
_____
_____
_____

Answer: _____
_____
_____
_____

Date   Doctor
__/__/__ _____
Question: _____
_____
_____
_____

Answer: _____
_____
_____
_____

Date   Doctor
__/__/__ _____
Question: _____
_____
_____
_____

Answer: _____
_____
_____
_____

Date   Doctor
__/__/__ _____
Question: _____
_____
_____
_____

Answer: _____
_____
_____
_____

Date   Doctor
__/__/__ _____
Question: _____
_____
_____
_____

Answer: _____
_____
_____
_____

Date   Doctor
__/__/__ _____
Question: _____
_____
_____
_____

Answer: _____
_____
_____
_____

Questions: Asked and Answered

Date   Doctor
__/__/__ _____
Question: _____

_____
_____
_____

Answer: _____

_____
_____
_____

Date   Doctor
__/__/__ _____
Question: _____

_____
_____
_____

Answer: _____

_____
_____
_____

Date   Doctor
__/__/__ _____
Question: _____

_____
_____
_____

Answer: _____

_____
_____
_____

Date   Doctor
__/__/__ _____
Question: _____

_____
_____
_____

Answer: _____

_____
_____
_____

Date   Doctor
__/__/__ _____
Question: _____

_____
_____
_____

Answer: _____

_____
_____
_____

Date   Doctor
__/__/__ _____
Question: _____

_____
_____
_____

Answer: _____

_____
_____
_____

Questions: Asked and Answered

Date   Doctor
__/__/__ _____
Question: _____
_____
_____
_____

Answer: _____
_____
_____
_____

Date   Doctor
__/__/__ _____
Question: _____
_____
_____
_____

Answer: _____
_____
_____
_____

Date   Doctor
__/__/__ _____
Question: _____
_____
_____
_____

Answer: _____
_____
_____
_____

Date   Doctor
__/__/__ _____
Question: _____
_____
_____
_____

Answer: _____
_____
_____
_____

Date   Doctor
__/__/__ _____
Question: _____
_____
_____
_____

Answer: _____
_____
_____
_____

Date   Doctor
__/__/__ _____
Question: _____
_____
_____
_____

Answer: _____
_____
_____
_____

Questions: Asked and Answered

Date   Doctor
_/_/_ _____
Question: _____
_____
_____
_____
Answer: _____
_____
_____
_____

Date   Doctor
_/_/_ _____
Question: _____
_____
_____
_____
Answer: _____
_____
_____
_____

Date   Doctor
_/_/_ _____
Question: _____
_____
_____
_____
Answer: _____
_____
_____
_____

Date   Doctor
_/_/_ _____
Question: _____
_____
_____
_____
Answer: _____
_____
_____
_____

Date   Doctor
_/_/_ _____
Question: _____
_____
_____
Answer: _____
_____
_____
_____

Date   Doctor
_/_/_ _____
Question: _____
_____
_____
Answer: _____
_____
_____
_____

Questions: Asked and Answered

Date   Doctor
__/__/__ _____
Question: _____
_____
_____
_____
_____

Answer: _____
_____
_____
_____

Date   Doctor
__/__/__ _____
Question: _____
_____
_____
_____
_____

Answer: _____
_____
_____
_____

Date   Doctor
__/__/__ _____
Question: _____
_____
_____
_____

Answer: _____
_____
_____
_____

Date   Doctor
__/__/__ _____
Question: _____
_____
_____
_____

Answer: _____
_____
_____
_____

Date   Doctor
__/__/__ _____
Question: _____
_____
_____

Answer: _____
_____
_____
_____

Date   Doctor
__/__/__ _____
Question: _____
_____
_____

Answer: _____
_____
_____
_____

Questions: Asked and Answered

Date   Doctor
__/__/__   _____
Question: _____

_____

_____

_____

Answer: _____

_____

_____

_____

Date   Doctor
__/__/__   _____
Question: _____

_____

_____

_____

Answer: _____

_____

_____

_____

Date   Doctor
__/__/__   _____
Question: _____

_____

_____

_____

Answer: _____

_____

_____

_____

Date   Doctor
__/__/__   _____
Question: _____

_____

_____

_____

Answer: _____

_____

_____

_____

Date   Doctor
__/__/__   _____
Question: _____

_____

_____

_____

Answer: _____

_____

_____

Date   Doctor
__/__/__   _____
Question: _____

_____

_____

_____

Answer: _____

_____

_____

Questions: Asked and Answered

Date   Doctor
__/__/__   _____
Question: _____
_____
_____
_____

Answer: _____
_____
_____
_____

Date   Doctor
__/__/__   _____
Question: _____
_____
_____
_____

Answer: _____
_____
_____
_____

Date   Doctor
__/__/__   _____
Question: _____
_____
_____
_____

Answer: _____
_____
_____
_____

Date   Doctor
__/__/__   _____
Question: _____
_____
_____
_____

Answer: _____
_____
_____
_____

Date   Doctor
__/__/__   _____
Question: _____
_____
_____
_____

Answer: _____
_____
_____
_____

Date   Doctor
__/__/__   _____
Question: _____
_____
_____
_____

Answer: _____
_____
_____
_____

Questions: Asked and Answered

Date   Doctor
__/__/__   _____
Question: _____
_____
_____
_____

Answer: _____
_____
_____
_____

Date   Doctor
__/__/__   _____
Question: _____
_____
_____
_____

Answer: _____
_____
_____
_____

Date   Doctor
__/__/__   _____
Question: _____
_____
_____
_____

Answer: _____
_____
_____
_____

Date   Doctor
__/__/__   _____
Question: _____
_____
_____
_____

Answer: _____
_____
_____
_____

Date   Doctor
__/__/__   _____
Question: _____
_____
_____
_____

Answer: _____
_____
_____
_____

Date   Doctor
__/__/__   _____
Question: _____
_____
_____
_____

Answer: _____
_____
_____
_____

ADDRESS

INFORMATION

"To every thing there is a season, and a time to every purpose under heaven."   Ecclesiastes 3:1

Address Information

Name_____ Phone ( )____/____home
Address_____ Phone ( )____/____office
City/State_____ Fax   ( )____/____
Zip Code_____ E-mail_____

Name_____ Phone ( )____/____home
Address_____ Phone ( )____/____office
City/State_____ Fax   ( )____/____
Zip Code_____ E-mail_____

Name_____ Phone ( )____/____home
Address_____ Phone ( )____/____office
City/State_____ Fax   ( )____/____
Zip Code_____ E-mail_____

Name_____ Phone ( )____/____home
Address_____ Phone ( )____/____office
City/State_____ Fax   ( )____/____
Zip Code_____ E-mail_____

Name_____ Phone ( )____/____home
Address_____ Phone ( )____/____office
City/State_____ Fax   ( )____/____
Zip Code_____ E-mail_____

Name_____ Phone ( )____/____home
Address_____ Phone ( )____/____office
City/State_____ Fax   ( )____/____
Zip Code_____ E-mail_____

Address Information

Name_____ Phone (____)____/____home
Address_____ Phone (____)____/____office
City/State_____ Fax (____)____/____
Zip Code_____ E-mail_____

Name_____ Phone (____)____/____home
Address_____ Phone (____)____/____office
City/State_____ Fax (____)____/____
Zip Code_____ E-mail_____

Name_____ Phone (____)____/____home
Address_____ Phone (____)____/____office
City/State_____ Fax (____)____/____
Zip Code_____ E-mail_____

Name_____ Phone (____)____/____home
Address_____ Phone (____)____/____office
City/State_____ Fax (____)____/____
Zip Code_____ E-mail_____

Name_____ Phone (____)____/____home
Address_____ Phone (____)____/____office
City/State_____ Fax (____)____/____
Zip Code_____ E-mail_____

Name_____ Phone (____)____/____home
Address_____ Phone (____)____/____office
City/State_____ Fax (____)____/____
Zip Code_____ E-mail_____

Address Information

Name_____   Phone (   )___/___home
Address_____   Phone (   )___/___office
City/State_____   Fax   (   )___/___
Zip Code_____   E-mail_____

Name_____   Phone (   )___/___home
Address_____   Phone (   )___/___office
City/State_____   Fax   (   )___/___
Zip Code_____   E-mail_____

Name_____   Phone (   )___/___home
Address_____   Phone (   )___/___office
City/State_____   Fax   (   )___/___
Zip Code_____   E-mail_____

Name_____   Phone (   )___/___home
Address_____   Phone (   )___/___office
City/State_____   Fax   (   )___/___
Zip Code_____   E-mail_____

Name_____   Phone (   )___/___home
Address_____   Phone (   )___/___office
City/State_____   Fax   (   )___/___
Zip Code_____   E-mail_____

Name_____   Phone (   )___/___home
Address_____   Phone (   )___/___office
City/State_____   Fax   (   )___/___
Zip Code_____   E-mail_____

Address Information

Name_____   Phone (   )____/____home
Address_____   Phone (   )____/____office
City/State_____   Fax   (   )____/____
Zip Code_____   E-mail_____

Name_____   Phone (   )____/____home
Address_____   Phone (   )____/____office
City/State_____   Fax   (   )____/____
Zip Code_____   E-mail_____

Name_____   Phone (   )____/____home
Address_____   Phone (   )____/____office
City/State_____   Fax   (   )____/____
Zip Code_____   E-mail_____

Name_____   Phone (   )____/____home
Address_____   Phone (   )____/____office
City/State_____   Fax   (   )____/____
Zip Code_____   E-mail_____

Name_____   Phone (   )____/____home
Address_____   Phone (   )____/____office
City/State_____   Fax   (   )____/____
Zip Code_____   E-mail_____

Name_____   Phone (   )____/____home
Address_____   Phone (   )____/____office
City/State_____   Fax   (   )____/____
Zip Code_____   E-mail_____

Address Information

Name_____	Phone ( )____/____home
Address_____	Phone ( )____/____office
City/State_____	Fax ( )____/____
Zip Code_____	E-mail_____

Name_____	Phone ( )____/____home
Address_____	Phone ( )____/____office
City/State_____	Fax ( )____/____
Zip Code_____	E-mail_____

Name_____	Phone ( )____/____home
Address_____	Phone ( )____/____office
City/State_____	Fax ( )____/____
Zip Code_____	E-mail_____

Name_____	Phone ( )____/____home
Address_____	Phone ( )____/____office
City/State_____	Fax ( )____/____
Zip Code_____	E-mail_____

Name_____	Phone ( )____/____home
Address_____	Phone ( )____/____office
City/State_____	Fax ( )____/____
Zip Code_____	E-mail_____

Name_____	Phone ( )____/____home
Address_____	Phone ( )____/____office
City/State_____	Fax ( )____/____
Zip Code_____	E-mail_____

Address Information

Name_____   Phone (   )____/____home
Address_____   Phone (   )____/____office
City/State_____   Fax   (   )____/____
Zip Code_____   E-mail_____

Name_____   Phone (   )____/____home
Address_____   Phone (   )____/____office
City/State_____   Fax   (   )____/____
Zip Code_____   E-mail_____

Name_____   Phone (   )____/____home
Address_____   Phone (   )____/____office
City/State_____   Fax   (   )____/____
Zip Code_____   E-mail_____

Name_____   Phone (   )____/____home
Address_____   Phone (   )____/____office
City/State_____   Fax   (   )____/____
Zip Code_____   E-mail_____

Name_____   Phone (   )____/____home
Address_____   Phone (   )____/____office
City/State_____   Fax   (   )____/____
Zip Code_____   E-mail_____

Name_____   Phone (   )____/____home
Address_____   Phone (   )____/____office
City/State_____   Fax   (   )____/____
Zip Code_____   E-mail_____

CALENDARS

"When pride comes, then comes disgrace, but with humility comes wisdom." Proverbs 11:2

2002

JANUARY	FEBRUARY	MARCH
S M T W T F S	S M T W T F S	S M T W T F S
1 2 3 4 5 6 7 8 9 10 11 12 13 14 15 16 17 18 19 20 21 22 23 24 25 26 27 28 29 30 31	1 2 3 4 5 6 7 8 9 10 11 12 13 14 15 16 17 18 19 20 21 22 23 24 25 26 27 28	1 2 3 4 5 6 7 8 9 10 11 12 13 14 15 16 17 18 19 20 21 22 23 24 25 26 27 28 29 30 31

APRIL	MAY	JUNE
S M T W T F S	S M T W T F S	S M T W T F S
1 2 3 4 5 6 7 8 9 10 11 12 13 14 15 16 17 18 19 20 21 22 23 24 25 26 27 28 29 30	1 2 3 4 5 6 7 8 9 10 11 12 13 14 15 16 17 18 19 20 21 22 23 24 25 26 27 28 29 30 31	1 2 3 4 5 6 7 8 9 10 11 12 13 14 15 16 17 18 19 20 21 22 23 24 25 26 27 28 29 30

JULY	AUGUST	SEPTEMBER
S M T W T F S	S M T W T F S	S M T W T F S
1 2 3 4 5 6 7 8 9 10 11 12 13 14 15 16 17 18 19 20 21 22 23 24 25 26 27 28 29 30 31	1 2 3 4 5 6 7 8 9 10 11 12 13 14 15 16 17 18 19 20 21 22 23 24 25 26 27 28 29 30 31	1 2 3 4 5 6 7 8 9 10 11 12 13 14 15 16 17 18 19 20 21 22 23 24 25 26 27 28 29 30

OCTOBER	NOVEMBER	DECEMBER
S M T W T F S	S M T W T F S	S M T W T F S
1 2 3 4 5 6 7 8 9 10 11 12 13 14 15 16 17 18 19 20 21 22 23 24 25 26 27 28 29 30 31	1 2 3 4 5 6 7 8 9 10 11 12 13 14 15 16 17 18 19 20 21 22 23 24 25 26 27 28 29 30	1 2 3 4 5 6 7 8 9 10 11 12 13 14 15 16 17 18 19 20 21 22 23 24 25 26 27 28 29 30 31

2003

JANUARY
S	M	T	W	T	F	S
		1	2	3	4	
5	6	7	8	9	10	11
12	13	14	15	16	17	18
19	20	21	22	23	24	25
26	27	28	29	30	31	

FEBRUARY
S	M	T	W	T	F	S
						1
2	3	4	5	6	7	8
9	10	11	12	13	14	15
16	17	18	19	20	21	22
23	24	25	26	27	28	

MARCH
S	M	T	W	T	F	S
						1
2	3	4	5	6	7	8
9	10	11	12	13	14	15
16	17	18	19	20	21	22
23	24	25	26	27	28	29
30	31					

APRIL
S	M	T	W	T	F	S
		1	2	3	4	5
6	7	8	9	10	11	12
13	14	15	16	17	18	19
20	21	22	23	24	25	26
27	28	29	30			

MAY
S	M	T	W	T	F	S
				1	2	3
4	5	6	7	8	9	10
11	12	13	14	15	16	17
18	19	20	21	22	23	24
25	26	27	28	29	30	31

JUNE
S	M	T	W	T	F	S
1	2	3	4	5	6	7
8	9	10	11	12	13	14
15	16	17	18	19	20	21
22	23	24	25	26	27	28
29	30					

JULY
S	M	T	W	T	F	S
		1	2	3	4	5
6	7	8	9	10	11	12
13	14	15	16	17	18	19
20	21	22	23	24	25	26
27	28	29	30	31		

AUGUST
S	M	T	W	T	F	S
					1	2
3	4	5	6	7	8	9
10	11	12	13	14	15	16
17	18	19	20	21	22	23
24	25	26	27	28	29	30
31						

SEPTEMBER
S	M	T	W	T	F	S
	1	2	3	4	5	6
7	8	9	10	11	12	13
14	15	16	17	18	19	20
21	22	23	24	25	26	27
28	29	30				

OCTOBER
S	M	T	W	T	F	S
			1	2	3	4
5	6	7	8	9	10	11
12	13	14	15	16	17	18
19	20	21	22	23	24	25
26	27	28	29	30	31	

NOVEMBER
S	M	T	W	T	F	S
						1
2	3	4	5	6	7	8
9	10	11	12	13	14	15
16	17	18	19	20	21	22
23	24	25	26	27	28	29
30						

DECEMBER
S	M	T	W	T	F	S
	1	2	3	4	5	6
7	8	9	10	11	12	13
14	15	16	17	18	19	20
21	22	23	24	25	26	27
28	29	30	31			

2004

JANUARY	FEBRUARY	MARCH
S M T W T F S	S M T W T F S	S M T W T F S
1 2 3 4 5 6 7 8 9 10 11 12 13 14 15 16 17 18 19 20 21 22 23 24 25 26 27 28 29 30 31	1 2 3 4 5 6 7 8 9 10 11 12 13 14 15 16 17 18 19 20 21 22 23 24 25 26 27 28 29	1 2 3 4 5 6 7 8 9 10 11 12 13 14 15 16 17 18 19 20 21 22 23 24 25 26 27 28 29 30 31

APRIL	MAY	JUNE
S M T W T F S	S M T W T F S	S M T W T F S
1 2 3 4 5 6 7 8 9 10 11 12 13 14 15 16 17 18 19 20 21 22 23 24 25 26 27 28 29 30	1 2 3 4 5 6 7 8 9 10 11 12 13 14 15 16 17 18 19 20 21 22 23 24 25 26 27 28 29 30 31	1 2 3 4 5 6 7 8 9 10 11 12 13 14 15 16 17 18 19 20 21 22 23 24 25 26 27 28 29 30

JULY	AUGUST	SEPTEMBER
S M T W T F S	S M T W T F S	S M T W T F S
1 2 3 4 5 6 7 8 9 10 11 12 13 14 15 16 17 18 19 20 21 22 23 24 25 26 27 28 29 30 31	1 2 3 4 5 6 7 8 9 10 11 12 13 14 15 16 17 18 19 20 21 22 23 24 25 26 27 28 29 30 31	1 2 3 4 5 6 7 8 9 10 11 12 13 14 15 16 17 18 19 20 21 22 23 24 25 26 27 28 29 30

OCTOBER	NOVEMBER	DECEMBER
S M T W T F S	S M T W T F S	S M T W T F S
1 2 3 4 5 6 7 8 9 10 11 12 13 14 15 16 17 18 19 20 21 22 23 24 25 26 27 28 29 30 31	1 2 3 4 5 6 7 8 9 10 11 12 13 14 15 16 17 18 19 20 21 22 23 24 25 26 27 28 29 30	1 2 3 4 5 6 7 8 9 10 11 12 13 14 15 16 17 18 19 20 21 22 23 24 25 26 27 28 29 30 31

2005

JANUARY	FEBRUARY	MARCH
S M T W T F S	S M T W T F S	S M T W T F S
1	1 2 3 4 5	1 2 3 4 5
2 3 4 5 6 7 8	6 7 8 9 10 11 12	6 7 8 9 10 11 12
9 10 11 12 13 14 15	13 14 15 16 17 18 19	13 14 15 16 17 18 19
16 17 18 19 20 21 22	20 21 22 23 24 25 26	20 21 22 23 24 25 26
23 24 25 26 27 28 29	27 28	27 28 29 30 31
30 31		

APRIL	MAY	JUNE
S M T W T F S	S M T W T F S	S M T W T F S
1 2	1 2 3 4 5 6 7	1 2 3 4
3 4 5 6 7 8 9	8 9 10 11 12 13 14	5 6 7 8 9 10 11
10 11 12 13 14 15 16	15 16 17 18 19 20 21	12 13 14 15 16 17 18
17 18 19 20 21 22 23	22 23 24 25 26 27 28	19 20 21 22 23 24 25
24 25 26 27 28 29 30	29 30 31	26 27 28 29 30 31

JULY	AUGUST	SEPTEMBER
S M T W T F S	S M T W T F S	S M T W T F S
1 2	1 2 3 4 5 6	1 2 3
3 4 5 6 7 8 9	7 8 9 10 11 12 13	4 5 6 7 8 9 10
10 11 12 13 14 15 16	14 15 16 17 18 19 20	11 12 13 14 15 16 17
17 18 19 20 21 22 23	21 22 23 24 25 26 27	18 19 20 21 22 23 24
24 25 26 27 28 29 30	28 29 30 31	25 26 27 28 29 30
31		

OCTOBER	NOVEMBER	DECEMBER
S M T W T F S	S M T W T F S	S M T W T F S
1	1 2 3 4 5	1 2 3
2 3 4 5 6 7 8	6 7 8 9 10 11 12	4 5 6 7 8 9 10
9 10 11 12 13 14 15	13 14 15 16 17 18 19	11 12 13 14 15 16 17
16 17 18 19 20 21 22	20 21 22 23 24 25 26	18 19 20 21 22 23 24
23 24 25 26 27 28 29	27 28 29 30	25 26 27 28 29 30 31
30 31		

161

Printed in the United States
1124600003B

9 781591 606901